THE SJOGREN'S SYNDROME HANDBOOK

An authoritative guide for patients

Edited by Elaine K. Harris

Medical Editors

Steven Carsons, M.D.

James J. Sciubba, D.M.D., Ph.D.

Norman Talal, M.D.

SJOGREN'S SYNDROME FOUNDATION INC.

Book design by Tom Pretnar

Library of Congress Cataloging in Publication Data

Harris, Elaine K., 1924–
    The Sjögren's Syndrome Handbook

    Bibliography:
    Includes index.
    1. Sjögren's syndrome.   2. Xerostomia (dry mouth).
    3. Keratoconjunctivitis sicca (dry eye).
    4. Rheumatoid arthritis.   5. Primary Sjögren's
    syndrome.   6. Secondary Sjögren's syndrome.
    7. Autoimmune disease.
    8. Exocrine glands.

I. Title.
WB 100.   WE 346
ISBN 0-9621157-0-3
Library of Congress Card Number 88-64215

PRINTED IN THE UNITED STATES OF AMERICA

To my husband Herbert Harris, for his love and understanding, his encouragement and support, his expertise and his patience. Without him, the Foundation and I could not have accomplished all we have done.

Elaine K. Harris

Acknowledgements

The publication of this book is the culmination of a dream.

It is a dream I shared with Bonnie Gustafsson and my husband Herbert Harris. Words cannot adequately describe the assistance, the intellectual and moral support, and the patience Herbert has contributed to the development of this book, through his participation in many different areas, his business acumen, his ability to get me to face reality, and his ability to keep his cool with a wife who could become quite "uptight," as well as overimmersed in the activities of the Sjogren's Syndrome Foundation (SSF) and the project at hand.

In 1985, Bonnie and I developed an outline for a Sjögren's syndrome handbook and guidelines for the authors to follow. We then proceeded to a discussion of authors for these important articles. We are most grateful to each of the authors (see Authors, pages ix–xiv) for so generously contributing these valuable articles without any remuneration, particularly since, as I have been told by many of the doctors, preparing an article for this kind of handbook was far more difficult than writing a paper for a professional audience (something they are accustomed to doing) or preparing a very simplistic presentation for a lay audience with no background on the subject.

From the conception of the idea straight through to publication, Dr. James J. Sciubba, the first Chairman of the Foundation's Medical Advisory Board (MAB), and Dr. Steven Carsons, also one of the original members of the MAB, have been participants in the development of the book. They, together with Dr. Norman Talal, current Chairman of our Medical Advisory Board, took on the difficult task of serving as Medical Editors of the book.

When Pat Costello Smith, our Manuscript Editor, agreed to take that role, I am sure she did not anticipate the tremendous amount of work that would be involved in this book, prepared by more than 30 authors and including several chapters by more than one author. Pat not only has handled her role with great skill and administrative competence, she has been for me a delight to work with.

Several people were most helpful in providing information about publishing and publishers, particularly Jesse Lehman, Dr. Irwin Mandel, and my very good friend Dr. Eugene Gottlieb, who introduced me to Tom Pretnar, who, as our book designer, ultimately guided me through the intricacies of publishing. Although the following doctors are not authors of chapters of the book, their helpful suggestions regarding content, as well as their review of various parts of the book, have been very valuable: Vincent P. deLuise, M.D., Philip Fox, D.D.S., Richard Furie, M.D., Jeffrey Gilbard, M.D., Ann Parke, M.D., Robert H. Phillips, Ph.D., Jan U. Prause, M.D., Ira Udell, M.D., and William E. Wright, D.D.S.

We are indebted to Dr. David Lamberts, coauthor of *Dry Eye Update*, and its publisher IOLAB for their permission to use the excellent illustrations from that book, and also to the Ciba-Geigy Corporation for permission to use a slide from *Clinical Symposia*, which so graphically shows the Sjögren's syndrome triad.

Publishing a book of this kind, with a fairly limited audience (after all, we are a "rare disorder"), needs financial backing. Many people have been generous in their support, but I must point out two very special contributions. One was from my cousins Eleanor and Arthur Feinberg, who, when I said I needed twenty $1,000 contributions or the equivalent thereof, gave the Foundation the first $1,000 contribution toward the development of the handbook. Dr. Norman Talal, who has played and is playing such a major role in spearheading research on Sjögren's syndrome, introduced me to Dr. George Koznetsky and his wife Ronya, President of the RGK Foundation, who showed great confidence in what we were trying to achieve and donated $5,000 toward the handbook. These two substantial contributions earmarked for the handbook gave us the cushion we needed to start.

Special memorial contributions were received from Lynne Murray, in memory of her mother May Schroeder; friends and family of the late Sueann Findo; Linda Harris and Jerrold Liebermann, in memory of Linda's grandmother Bertha Kirschbaum; and friends and family of the late Janet Davis.

The special efforts of Gracie Blanton and Vera Gatanos were responsible for the contributions from the Armed Forces auxiliaries, the Air Forces Officers' Wives Club, the Fort Belvoir Enlisted Wives Club, and the Fort Belvoir Officers' Wives Club. Other significant contributions earmarked for the handbook were received from Alcon Laboratories, Inc.; Allergan Pharmaceuticals, Inc.; the late Bertha Kirschbaum; and the Kraus-Perlstein Foundation of Brith Sholom.

Not to be forgotten and far too numerous to list individually are the many members and friends who offered small but important suggestions, and the contributors who have supported and continue to support the many other educational activities of the Sjogren's Syndrome Foundation.

To each of you, for your confidence and support in helping to bring forth this most important book, I thank you.

Elaine K. Harris
November 30, 1988

Authors

Andrew P. Andonopoulos, M.D.
Consultant Rheumatologist
Department of Internal Medicine
School of Medicine
University of Ioannina
Ioannina, GREECE

Charles S. Baraf, M.D.
Assistant Professor
Health Sciences Center
State University of New York at Stony Brook
Chief of Dermatology
Long Island Jewish Medical Center
New Hyde Park, NY

Kenneth Berk, O.D.
Optometrist in general practice
New York, NY

Jill P. Buyon, M.D.
Assistant Professor
New York University Medical Center
Associate Attending Physician
Hospital for Joint Diseases
Orthopaedic Institute
New York, NY

Steven Carsons, M.D.
Assistant Professor of Medicine
Health Sciences Center
State University of New York at Stony Brook
Chief of Division of Rheumatology,
Clinical Immunology, and Allergy
Winthrop University Hospital
Mineola, NY

Troy E. Daniels, D.D.S, M.S.
Professor of Oral Medicine
Chairman of Oral Pathology
Director, Sjögren's Syndrome Clinic
School of Dentistry
University of California, San Francisco
San Francisco, CA

R. Linsy Farris, M.D.
Professor of Clinical Ophthalmology
College of Physicians and Surgeons
Columbia University
Attending Physician
Cornea and External Eye Diseases
Edward S. Harkness Eye Institute
Columbia-Presbyterian Medical Center
Director of Ophthalmology
Harlem Hospital Medical Center
New York, NY

Mark Flapan, Ph.D.
Psychologist in private practice
President, Scleroderma Society, Inc.
New York, NY

Robert I. Fox, M.D., Ph.D.
Adjunct Assistant Member
Department of Basic and Clinical Research
Scripps Clinic and Research Foundation
La Jolla, CA

Mitchell Friedlaender, M.D.
Adjunct Associate Member
Division of Opthalmology
Scripps Clinic and Research Foundation
La Jolla, CA

Bonnie A. Gustafsson, B.A.
Board of Directors
Sjogren's Syndrome Foundation
Member, American Medical Writers Association

Elaine K. Harris, M.A.
President and Founder
Sjogren's Syndrome Foundation
Editor, *The Moisture Seekers Newsletter*

Francis V. Howell, D.D.S.
Head, Oral Pathology Division
Pathology Medical Laboratories
La Jolla, CA

David A. Isenberg, M.D.
Consultant Rheumatologist
Bloomsbury Rheumatology Unit
University College and
Middlesex Hospital Schools of Medicine
London, ENGLAND

Eden Kalman, M.A., R.D.
Adjunct Instructor
New York University
Nutritionist
Assistant Director, Food Services
Hospital for Special Surgery
New York, NY

Robert J. Kassan, M.D.
Rheumatologist, Pompano Beach, FL
President, Southeast Florida Branch
Arthritis Foundation

Stuart S. Kassan, M.D.
Associate Clinical Professor of Medicine
University of Colorado
Health Sciences Center
Medical Director, Rehabilitation Center
Lutheran Medical Center
Denver, CO

Seymour Katz, M.D.
Clinical Associate Professor of Medicine
Cornell University Medical College
Attending Physician
North Shore University Hospital
Manhasset, NY
Long Island Jewish Medical Center
New Hyde Park, NY
St. Francis Hospital
Roslyn, NY

Paul B. Lang, M.D.
Clinical Associate Professor of Medicine
Cornell University Medical College
Chief of Allergy
North Shore University Hospital
Manhasset, NY

Joan Levy, M.A., C.C.C. in Speech
Chief of Speech Pathology
Long Island Jewish Medical Center
New Hyde Park, NY

Daniel M. Libby, M.D.
Clinical Associate Professor of Medicine
Cornell University Medical College
Associate Attending Physician
New York Hospital
New York, NY

Irwin D. Mandel, M.D.
Professor of Dentistry and Director
Center for Clinical Research in Dentistry
School of Dental and Oral Surgery
Columbia University
New York, NY

Haralampos M. Moutsopoulos, M.D.
Professor and Chairman
Department of Internal Medicine
Medical School
University of Ioannina
Ioannina, GREECE

Kenneth Nyer, M.D.
Clinical Instructor of Internal Medicine
Cornell University Medical College
Attending Physician
North Shore University Hospital
Manhasset, NY

Roger Miles Rose, M.D.
Associate Professor of Otolaryngology
New York University College of Medicine
Attending Physician
New York University Medical Center
Lenox Hill Hospital
New York, NY

James J. Sciubba, D.M.D., Ph.D.
Professor of Oral Biology and Pathology
School of Dental Medicine
Health Sciences Center
State University of New York at Stony Brook
Chairman, Department of Dentistry
Long Island Jewish Medical Center
New Hyde Park, NY

Michael L. Snaith, M.D.
Consultant Rheumatologist
Bloomsbury Health Authority
Senior Clinical Lecturer
University College and
Middlesex Schools of Medicine
London, ENGLAND

Harry Spiera, M.D.
Clinical Professor of Medicine
Chief, Division of Rheumatology
Mount Sinai Medical Center
New York, NY

Norman Talal, M.D.
Professor of Medicine and Microbiology
Head, Division of Clinical Immunology and Rheumatology
University of Texas Health Science Center at San Antonio and
Audie Murphy Memorial Veterans Administration Hospital
San Antonio, TX

John J. Willems, M.D.
Associate Clinical Professor
University of California, San Diego
Director, Vulvar Disease Clinic
Scripps Clinic and Research Foundation
La Jolla, CA

Contents

Part III Extraglandular Involvement

Part IV Caring for Yourself

Appendices

Preface

This book is very special. It represents a unique cooperation, as well as an understanding, between the medical specialists who treat Sjögren's syndrome (SS) and the Sjogren's Syndrome Foundation Inc. (SSF), an organization dedicated to helping SS patients live more comfortably with this chronic, debilitating, painful, and frustrating disease.

The fact that you have this handbook to read and reread, to show to family and friends, so that they will understand your pains and your frustrations, is a tribute to the doctors who responded to my plea to develop patient information materials that would help us understand what was happening to our bodies and, although there is not yet a cure, what we can do to make ourselves more comfortable.

When I was first diagnosed as having Sjögren's syndrome, after a year of having gone from doctor to doctor in an effort to find out what was wrong with me—why I hurt all over, ran a low-grade fever almost continually, had dry, painful eyes, nostrils that were full of sores, white spots on my palate, excruciatingly painful sore throats, armpits that were convex, rather than concave, due to swollen lymph glands, and a deep-seated earache, to mention only some of my symptoms—there was no readily available patient information to explain the illness and no mutual aid group to turn to. How fortunate for you that, thanks to the Sjogren's Syndrome Foundation, this is no longer true. Appendix C contains a history of the Foundation from its birth as a self-help group that I started at the Long Island Jewish Medical Center (LIJMC) to its development as the world's leading organization for patient information on Sjögren's syndrome.

In 1986, Dr. Norman Talal asked me to write a chapter on "The Patient's Perspective" for the medical text that he, Dr. H. M. Moutsopoulos, and Dr. S. S. Kassan were editing, *Sjögren's Syndrome: Clinical and Immunological Aspects* (published in 1987 by Springer-Verlag). My comments included the following:

Sjögren's syndrome patients have several problems unique to their disease:

(1) The difficulty in achieving a diagnosis due to:

(a) the discrete, seemingly unrelated symptoms. How many patients would think of telling their ophthalmologist that they are also suffering from a dry mouth? Or their dentist that they have dry eyes that burn, are glued together, and 'shut down' at night?

(b) the lack of awareness in general practitioners about SS and its manifestations;

(c) the great fluctuations in their symptoms and signs.

(2) The lack of knowledge by many physicians treating SS patients regarding practical tips to help many patients live and function more comfortably.

(3) The impracticality of a doctor being able to take the time to explain the ramifications and background of this disease to a patient, because of the vast amount of time involved and the lack of reference material for patients.

(4) The inability to communicate with other patients, because so few people know about SS; in fact, many who have Sjögren's are not aware they have it.

(5) The need for coordinated medical care so that:

(a) patients do not have to run from place to place to see the doctors caring for them;

(b) the physicians involved in the patient's care can com-

municate knowledgeably and quickly, making a group evaluation and recommendations for treatment not only feasible, but very practicable.

It is almost 1989. Do these problems still exist? For some of you, the answer will be an emphatic "Yes." For many others, however, the answer will be "No" or "It's not as bad as it was." Public and medical awareness about Sjögren's syndrome are definitely on the increase. The February, 1989, issue of the *FDA Consumer,* the official magazine of the U. S. Food and Drug Administration, will feature an article on Sjögren's syndrome.

In January, 1989, there will be a most important conference, sponsored by the National Institute of Arthritis, Musculoskeletal, and Skin Diseases and the Arthritis and Musculoskeletal Diseases Interagency Coordinating Committee of the National Institutes of Health (NIH) on "The Many Faces of Sjögren's Syndrome." This conference will present the state of the art in diagnosis and treatment of Sjögren's syndrome to primary care physicians, dentists, and other health care professionals. It means that, at long last, the latest medical information on SS will be available for the nonspecialist—for the doctors we see when we first start to feel ill. The proceedings of this important conference will be available. (Information on obtaining them will appear in *The Moisture Seekers Newsletter.)*

The need for coordinated medical care still exists, but as the identifiable Sjögren's population is increasing, so, too, are the medical centers trying to improve their services to SS patients by developing a team approach for treating them, or at least by having some kind of coordinated SS care among the major medical specialties involved (medicine, ophthalmology, and dentistry).

Will there ever be a cure for Sjögren's syndrome? We certainly hope so. Researchers continue to probe for the secrets that regulate the immune system. A disease cannot be cured until what causes it (the etiology) is definitely understood. Meanwhile, many dedicated physicians and dentists are working on treatments—to find artificial tears (no one tear will help all of us); to find an almost tasteless oral lubricant that truly lubricates the interior of our mouths; to find a medication that will combat the feelings of exhaustion and malaise we have, in addition to our dry eyes, dry mouth, dry vagina, etc.

Others are working on devices to stimulate secretions. Many of us have heard about bromhexine, a medication widely used in Europe for the treatment of Sjögren's syndrome. Work is underway in the United States to test its safety and efficacy as a treatment for Sjögren's syndrome. Doctors are working on a special form of cyclosporin, which initial tests have shown stimulates tear production. A new electronic device recently appeared on the market (see *FDA Consumer,* October, 1988) to stimulate salivary production. Work is being done to develop a saliva that will stimulate the particular salivary gland that has lost its function.

Recent studies have shown that the drug Plaquenil may be effective in relieving the systemic symptoms of SS. Someone is working on a device to supply warm, moisturized air to the nose. In a few years, when this book is reprinted, I hope there will be reports on the positive results of these developing treatments.

You will learn much as you read this book. Following the Introduction by Dr. Talal, you will note that the body of the book is organized into four main sections: Part I, An Overview, which explains what Sjögren's syndrome is, its causes, and how it is diagnosed; Part II, Glandular Involvement, which covers the organs directly affected by the exocrine (mucous-secreting) glands; Part III, Extraglandular Involvement, which covers the organs that do not have mucous-secreting glands; and Part IV, Caring for Yourself, which covers daily living, including coping with a chronic disease, nutrition, tips for travel, etc.

The Glossary (Appendix A) explains scientific terms used in the text. You will want to refer to it, if you come across a medical term with which you are unfamiliar. Since one of the most frequent requests we receive at the SSF office is, "How can I get moisture chamber glasses?," instructions for the optician to follow are in Appendix B. Making them requires practice, skill, and a great deal of patience by both the optician fitting them and the patient who will be wearing them, who must sit patiently as each minute adjustment is made. Many people have expressed an interest in the history of the Sjogren's Syndrome Foundation. It is the "last, but not least" section of the Appendices.

The Medical Advisory Board of the Sjogren's Syndrome Foundation deliberated on the issue of including a list of treatment centers in this book. Because these centers and the services they offer are so varied and subject to change, the Medical Advisory Board decided that such a list should not be included.

If this book and the Foundation had both been available when I was first diagnosed as having Sjögren's syndrome, I would not have felt the desperate need that I did to start that first group at the Long Island Jewish Medical Center in 1983. Yes, with chapters and contact leaders of the SSF all over the world, and now a handbook filled with important information, things are definitely improving for the SS patient. We are not alone. You can pick up a phone and talk with another person who has SS, sharing your concerns and your improvements. More and more doctors are now interested in SS and knowledgeable about how to properly treat people who have it. More and more people are discovering that they have SS. And more and more doctors are becoming involved in research to find the cause and a cure for SS.

Will SS be conquered in our time? I don't know. But there is hope. Meanwhile, read and learn. You will find that knowing about your Sjögren's syndrome will help you to live more comfortably with it. It has helped me and it will help you.

Elaine K. Harris
November 16, 1988

Introduction for the Patient

At the outset, I would like to congratulate the founders, volunteers, and sustainers of the Sjogren's Syndrome Foundation, also known as the Moisture Seekers, for their success in establishing, developing, and maintaining this extremely important organization. By your very existence, you make my job easier as a physician and medical scientist vitally interested in Sjögren's syndrome (SS). The physicians who work on SS and the patients who endure it wish you Godspeed for your continued success.

Sjögren's syndrome is named for the Swedish ophthalmologist Henrik Sjögren, who prior to World War II described a triad of symptoms—dry eyes, dry mouth, and rheumatoid arthritis—in patients consulting him for their eye complaints. The disease had been described earlier, in the last half of the nineteenth century, by other European physicians. Because Sjögren, who died at an advanced age in 1987, wrote extensively about his clinical experience, the condition bears his name.

An alternative name for Sjögren's syndrome is *autoimmune exocrinopathy,* which more aptly describes the immune system's attack on the exocrine glands—salivary, lacrimal (tear), and other moisture-secreting glands. In SS and other autoimmune diseases, the body's defense or immune system mistakes some of the patient's own tissues as foreign invaders. In SS, the immune system targets the moisture-secreting glands, most noticeably the salivary and tear glands. The resultant dryness causes mouth and eye discomfort. In women, SS may affect the moisture-producing Bartholin's glands, leading to vaginal dryness.

Sjögren's syndrome is a systemic disease that can involve many organs in the body, including the lung and kidney. Accordingly, several medical and dental specialists may be needed to manage and treat a patient with this illness. Since half of SS patients have arthritis, rheumatologists are generally the best trained and most experienced to deal with this disease. If the rheumatologist has had a broad exposure to clinical immunology as part of his or her training, so much the better.

Frequent dental checkups by a competent dentist and regular visits to an ophthalmologist (a physician specializing in eye disorders) are important parts of the team approach to optimal patient management. This will help assure the least disability from the disease and best possible outcome.

Many patients do fairly well. The vast majority lead productive lives. Symptoms are often controlled with eye drops and arthritis medications, as needed. Mouth dryness continues to be a major source of patient discomfort, but researchers are working hard on this problem. An optimistic outlook and faith in the future will help immeasurably in achieving the therapeutic goal of living as normal a life as possible.

What of the future? Let me assure you that recent advances in medical science and biotechnology will, I believe, revolutionize our understanding and ability to treat many chronic diseases, including Sjögren's syndrome. I promise my medical students that, one day soon, they will have a new array of drugs, called immunomodulators, in their black bags to treat autoimmune diseases.

Sjögren's syndrome will be conquered, hopefully in our lifetime. Your involvement in the Sjogren's Syndrome Foundation can bring that day closer, for you are not only a patient support group, you are resources who can go out and lobby for the research funds necessary to find the cause and cure of your disease.

Norman Talal
May 11, 1988

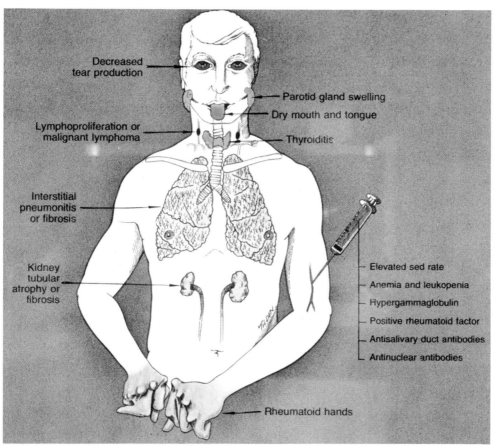

Systemic manifestions that may be indicative of Sjögren's syndrome.

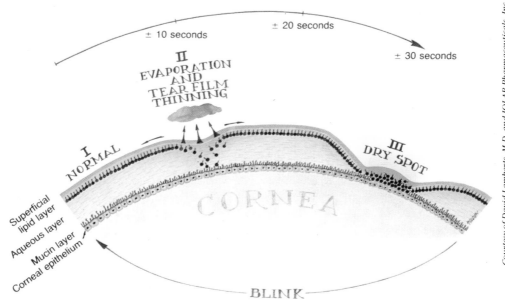

The tear film is composed of three layers — lipid, aqueous and mucin — resting on the cornea. Localized excessive rate of evaporation produces tear film thinning and eventually dry spots.

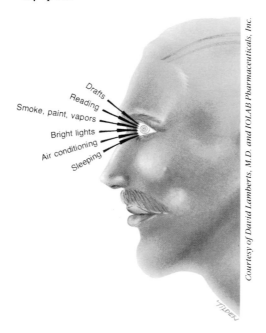

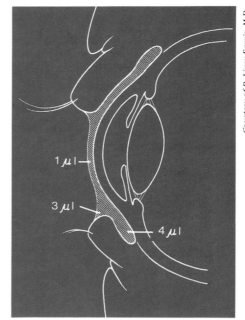

Evaporation may exceed the rate of tear production and produce a dry eye. Drafts, reading, fumes, bright lights, air conditioning and sleeping influence evaporative loss of tears from one extreme to another.

The small volume of tears on the exposed surface of the eye (1 µl) requires frequent replenishment by secretion, blinking and spreading of the tears in the inferior marginal tear strip (3 µl) and tears from behind the lids (4 µl).

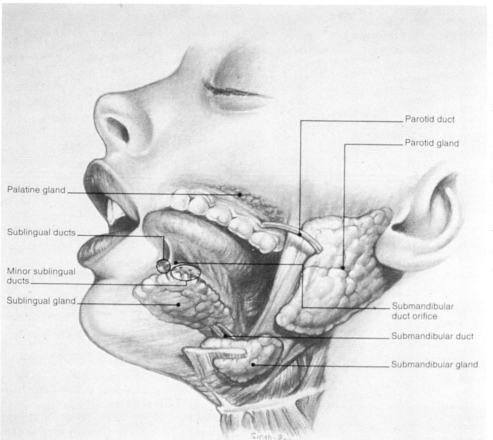

Parotid duct

Parotid gland

Palatine gland

Sublingual ducts

Minor sublingual
ducts

Sublingual gland

Submandibular
duct orifice

Submandibular duct

Submandibular gland

The salivary glands.

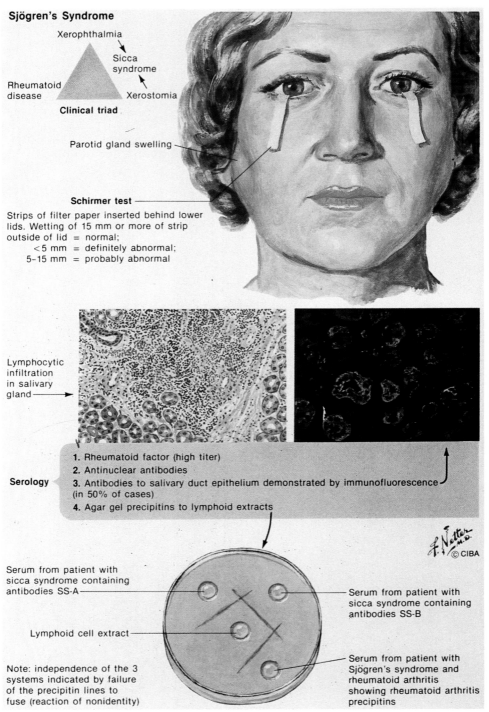

Sjögren's Syndrome

Xerophthalmia

Sicca syndrome

Rheumatoid disease

Xerostomia

Clinical triad

Parotid gland swelling

Schirmer test
Strips of filter paper inserted behind lower lids. Wetting of 15 mm or more of strip outside of lid = normal;
 <5 mm = definitely abnormal;
 5–15 mm = probably abnormal

Lymphocytic infiltration in salivary gland

Serology
1. Rheumatoid factor (high titer)
2. Antinuclear antibodies
3. Antibodies to salivary duct epithelium demonstrated by immunofluorescence (in 50% of cases)
4. Agar gel precipitins to lymphoid extracts

Serum from patient with sicca syndrome containing antibodies SS-A

Serum from patient with sicca syndrome containing antibodies SS-B

Lymphoid cell extract

Note: independence of the 3 systems indicated by failure of the precipitin lines to fuse (reaction of nonidentity)

Serum from patient with Sjögren's syndrome and rheumatoid arthritis showing rheumatoid arthritis precipitins

The triad of xerostomia (dry mouth), keratoconjunctivitis sicca (dry eye) and a rheumatoid disease constitutes Sjögren's syndrome. Xerostomia and keratoconjunctivitis alone constitute the sicca syndrome or sicca complex (Primary SS).

Part I

An Overview

1

What is Sjögren's Syndrome?

Norman Talal, M.D.

Sjögren's syndrome (SS) is a chronic inflammatory disease characterized by the sicca complex (decreased tears and saliva) and resulting in keratoconjunctivitis sicca (KCS or dry eyes) and xerostomia (dry mouth). (The symptoms of SS are outlined in Table 1.)

Scientists think of the immune system as the body's way of defending itself against disease. Immune system cells, called lymphocytes and plasma cells, protect the body by killing foreign organisms, such as viruses and bacteria. In Sjögren's syndrome and several other autoimmune diseases, however, the immune system mistakes the body's own cells as alien invaders. We call this process *autoimmunity*.

In patients with SS, lymphocytes selectively destroy and replace moisture-producing glandular tissue, most noticeably the salivary and lacrimal glands, causing them to lose their ability to produce saliva and tears.

Any material the body recognizes as foreign is called an *antigen*. Antigens provoke the immune system to produce *antibodies*, blood proteins that help kill these organisms. The measles virus, for example, stimulates the immune system to generate antibodies against measles.

In autoimmune diseases, the immune system, recognizing the body's own tissues as antigens, begins to make *autoantibodies* or antibodies that attack these tissues and organs as if they were foreign. No one yet knows why. This attack is much like the rejection of foreign tissue that occurs after skin or kidney is grafted from one person to another.

In Sjögren's syndrome, the exocrine or moisture-secreting glands become the targeted organs, so the disease is also called *autoimmune exocrinopathy*. Individuals with SS make certain autoantibodies, such as rheumatoid factor (RF) and antinuclear antibodies (ANAs), which can be detected in their blood.

No longer considered a medical rarity, Sjögren's syndrome is seen in 15% of the 2.1 million patients with rheumatoid arthritis (RA) in the United States. Moreover, for every person in whom the disease is associated with RA, there is probably another in whom it is not. And many cases go undetected, since symptoms may be mild and easily overlooked.

Only 50% of patients referred for Sjögren's syndrome actually have an autoimmune disease. Oral and ocular dryness frequently have other causes, such as sarcoidosis, endocrine disorders, anxiety-depression syndromes, and drugs that affect the parasympathetic nervous system.

DIAGNOSING SJOGREN'S SYNDROME

A diagnosis of Sjögren's syndrome is made when two out of the following three cardinal features are present: (1) definite KCS (dry eyes); (2) positive lip biopsy, confirming immune cells or lymphocytes as the cause for the dry mouth; (3) an associated extraglandular connective tissue (joints, skin, muscles) disorder, such as rheumatoid arthritis or systemic lupus erythematosus (SLE), commonly known as lupus.

Primary Sjögren's syndrome requires both (1) and (2) above, whereas secondary Sjögren's syndrome requires (3) plus either (1) or (2). There are immunogenetic, autoantibody, and clinical differences between these two categories of SS. (Table 2.)

More than 90% of Sjögren's syndrome patients are women, whose mean age is 50 years. SS occurs in all races and in children. Patients most commonly consult a physician because of: (1) the slowly progressive development of dry eyes and/or dry mouth in an individual who already has chronic rheumatoid arthritis; or (2) the more rapid development of a severe oral and ocular dryness, often accompanied by parotid gland swelling in an otherwise well person. (The parotid salivary glands are located near the ears. These are the glands that swell when an individual has mumps.)

Although fatigue and a "hurt-all-over" feeling are not measurable, these symptoms are frequently reported by individuals with SS.

OCULAR SYMPTOMS

About 50% of patients with KCS or dry eyes have additional features of Sjögren's syndrome. The most common ocular complaint is a sensation, described as "gritty" or "sandy," of a foreign body in the eye. Other symptoms include burning and accumulation of thick, ropy strands of mucus at the inner corners of the eyelids, particularly on awakening. Individuals with KCS also experience decreased tearing, redness, photosensitivity, eye fatigue, itching, and a "filmy" sensation that interferes with vision. They complain of eye discomfort and difficulty in reading or in watching television. Inability to cry is not a common complaint and lacrimal (tear) gland enlargement does not occur very often.

SALIVARY SYMPTOMS

The distressing manifestations of dry mouth include: difficulty with chewing, swallowing, and speaking; adherence of food to the buccal (cheek) surfaces; abnormalities of taste or smell; fissures (cracks) of the tongue, mucous membranes, and lips, particularly at the corners of the mouth; frequent ingestion of liquids, especially at mealtimes; and rampant dental decay.

These patients are unable to swallow a dry cracker or toast without ingesting fluids, and they express displeasure at the suggestion. This symptom has been called the "cracker sign." Individuals with dry mouth may carry bottles of water or other lubricants with them. They may awaken at night for sips of water. The dentist may notice that fillings are loosening or breaking down before their usual life span.

Dryness may also involve the nose, throat, larynx, and tracheobronchial tree and may lead to epistaxis (nosebleed), hoarseness, recurrent otitis media (inflammation of the middle ear), bronchitis, or pneumonia.

Half of the patients have enlargement of the parotid glands, often recurrent and symmetrical and sometimes accompanied by fever, tenderness, or erythema (redness of the skin). Complicating infections are rare. Rapid fluctuations in gland size are not unusual, but a particularly hard or nodular gland may suggest a tumor, usually noncancerous.

SYSTEMIC OR EXTRAGLANDULAR SYMPTOMS

The arthritis of Sjögren's syndrome resembles classic rheumatoid arthritis in many of its features. Dry eyes develop in about 10% to 15% of patients with RA. Patients with sicca complex (dry eyes/dry mouth) may experience joint pain and morning stiffness, without joint deformity. Fluctuations in the arthritis are not accompanied by similar fluctuations in the sicca complex symptoms.

Patients frequently experience skin dryness, vaginal dryness, and allergic drug eruptions. Red spots, called purpura, sometimes preceded by itching, may come and go on the legs. Nephritis (kidney inflammation) rarely develops and should suggest coexisting lupus.

Severe muscle weakness may be an early symptom leading to a diagnosis of polymyositis, another connective tissue disorder. Muscle tenderness is rare. Involvement of peripheral nerves, those outside the central nervous system (CNS), may cause symptoms of numbness or tingling. CNS (brain and spinal cord) involvement is associated with vasculitis (inflammation of a blood vessel), but this is rare.

IMMUNOGENIC ASPECTS

Scientific advances in immunogenetics (the study of genetic factors that control the immune response) and the detection of specific autoantibodies have helped distinguish primary from secondary Sjögren's syndrome. In primary SS, sicca symptoms are present, but there is no rheumatoid arthritis or other connective tissue disease. In secondary SS, the patient has dry eyes and/or dry mouth and a connective tissue disease as well.

Researchers have found that patients with rheumatoid arthritis and secondary Sjögren's syndrome, like patients with RA alone, are positive for HLA-DR4. HLA-DR4 is the name of a gene determining a particular type of body tissue. Tissue typing tests, originally developed during organ transplant research, are similar to tests that determine blood type.

Patients with primary Sjögren's syndrome, on the other hand, are often positive for HLA-B8-DR3. In this regard, they are somewhat like people with lupus.

Despite genetic associations, the possibility of inheriting Sjögren's syndrome is not very strong. If you have SS, it certainly does not mean your children necessarily will have the disease.

Positive tests for antinuclear antibodies are common in several rheumatic diseases. However, because specific ANAs (autoantibodies that react with nuclear antigens or antigens to the protein material released from cells) are different in each, these tests help distinguish primary from secondary SS.

Autoantibodies called SS-B or La are found in the blood of the majority of patients with primary Sjögren's syndrome. They are also found in lupus patients, particularly when SS is present. Autoantibodies known as SS-A or Ro are also associated with primary SS, but may occur in lupus as well.

TABLE 1.   SIGNS/SYMPTOMS OF SJOGREN'S SYNDROME

ORAL/SALIVARY SYMPTOMS:
- dry mouth
- "cracker sign"
- burning oral mucous membranes
- parotid gland hardening or enlargement
- dental caries
- inflamed oral mucosa
- dry, sticky oral mucosal surfaces
- reduced stimulated and unstimulated salivary flow rates
- inflamed salivary glands found in minor biopsy
- increased frequency of chronic yeast infections

OCULAR SIGNS/SYMPTOMS:
- foreign body sensation
- inability to tear
- abnormal visual intolerance to light
- reduced unanesthetized Schirmer test
- decreased tear breakup time
- twisted filaments of mucus on the surface of the cornea (the transparent "watch crystal" layer on the front of the eye)
- decreased tears
- characteristic rose bengal test
  (Eye tests for SS are discussed in Chapter 4.)

SYSTEMIC OR EXTRAGLANDULAR SIGNS/SYMPTOMS:
- rheumatoid arthritis or other connective tissue disease
- fatigue
- fever
- infiltration of autoantibodies in the lungs
- kidney, muscle, nerve, and liver disorders
- abnormal globulins (a class of proteins) in the blood
- excess gamma globulin
- rheumatoid factor (RF), antinuclear antibodies (ANAs), Ro/SS-A, La/SS-B autoantibodies

TABLE 2. DISTINGUISHING CHARACTERISTICS OF PRIMARY AND SECONDARY SS

PRIMARY SS:

- definite keratoconjunctivitis sicca (KCS or dry eyes) and a positive lip biopsy, confirming immune cells as the cause for dry mouth, with no evidence of other underlying rheumatic disease
- HLA-B8-DR3 positive
- antinuclear antibodies to Ro/SS-A or La/SS-B

SECONDARY SS:

- definite KCS and/or positive lip biopsy, plus evidence of accompanying rheumatoid arthritis (RA) or other connective tissue disease
- immunogenetic and serologic findings of accompanying disease, for example, HLA-DR4 positive, if patient has rheumatoid arthritis

2

Causes

Robert I. Fox, M.D. Ph.D.
Francis V. Howell, D.D.S.
Mitchell Friedlaender, M.D.

Sjögren's syndrome (SS) is characterized by dry eyes and dry mouth due to infiltration of the lacrimal (tear) and salivary glands by lymphocytes (a type of white blood cell involved in protecting the body from viral and bacterial infections). The blood of SS patients also contains antibodies (substances in the blood that are normally made in response to infections); these antibodies are directed against normal components of the cell. For many years, these observations have led investigators to speculate that SS is an *autoimmune* disorder; in other words, the body appears to be attacking itself. The factors triggering this autoimmunity remain poorly understood. However, it appears that genetic factors (traits inherited from parents) in SS patients and infectious agents work together to fool the immune system and to generate an autoimmune attack on the glands. In this regard, the mechanisms of pathogenesis may be similar to those proposed for diseases such as diabetes, which affects the gland in the pancreas, or thryroiditis, in which immune system cells (lymphocytes) destroy the thyroid gland in the presence of autoantibodies.

When trying to discover the cause(s) of a particular disease such as SS, the first step is to carefully define the clinical disorder. Otherwise, several different disease processes might be included under the same "label," obscuring the search for the most important factors. Although a 1986 international conference on SS in Copenhagen provided an initial step in clarification, there are still no uniformly accepted criteria for diagnosis. It is likely that this debate on diagnostic criteria will continue until specific genetic and environmental factors involved in SS are defined, thus serving as a definitive basis for diagnosis.

SCIENTIFIC STUDIES

Historically, Sjögren's syndrome was first described in 1892 by Johannes von Mikulicz, a Polish surgeon. However, because the term "Mikulicz syndrome" was subsequently used to describe several other disease processes, it became meaningless. Today, scientists are trying to define SS more carefully, avoiding the mistake of lumping several processes into one disease classification.

Although Henrik Sjögren first reported characteristic eye findings in his rheumatoid arthritis patients in 1932, his research was not generally appreciated until it was rediscovered in 1953 by two American researchers, William Morgan and Benjamin Castleman. Since then, many studies have been published about the clinical and laboratory features of SS patients.

The key features currently used for diagnosis of Sjögren's syndrome include: (1) dry eyes with findings of keratoconjunctivitis sicca on ophthalmologic exam; (2) dry mouth with characteristic findings within minor salivary glands; (3) evidence of a systemic autoimmune disease, as indicated by the presence of circulating autoantibodies; and (4) absence of other disorders, such as lymphoma, sarcoidosis, infection, or different diseases that can mimic Sjögren's syndrome.

In addition to the eyes and mouth, SS patients can have involvement of other organs, including the lungs, kidneys, thyroid, and nerves. Thus, the finding of eye and mouth symptoms must alert the physician to search for other possible tissue involvement.

The frequency of certain symptoms associated with Sjögren's

syndrome has varied greatly among different medical centers. For example, neurologic findings of multiple sclerosis and Alzheimer's disease were reported with high frequency at one center, but were not found to be significantly increased at other centers. It is possible that these differences result from varying criteria that are used to diagnose "SS."

OTHER CAUSES OF DRYNESS

Before turning to the specific genetic and environmental factors underlying Sjögren's syndrome, several pitfalls in attempts to classify patients with dry mouth and dry eye problems must be pointed out. First, salivary and lacrimal gland functions decrease as a normal part of aging. Autopsy studies show that over 40% of older patients have significant lymphocytic infiltrates in their salivary glands. Under microscopic examination, however, the specific appearance of these infiltrates is slightly different than that seen in younger patients who have been diagnosed as SS.

Certain degenerative disorders, such as Alzheimer's disease, are relatively common in the elderly, occurring in up to 5% of this population. Since older patients frequently have dry eyes and dry mouth, also, it is not surprising to find older individuals who have both Alzheimer's disease and dry eyes simply by coincidence of two common diseases in the same person. Thus, it would be incorrect to conclude that SS causes Alzheimer's disease or that younger SS patients have an increased risk of developing Alzheimer's disease.

Second, the characteristic appearance of lymphocytic infiltrates surrounding blood vessels on salivary gland biopsy is not specific to Sjögren's syndrome. A similar pattern of lymphocytic infiltrates occurs throughout the body in many autoimmune diseases. While the biopsy of salivary glands yields a convenient site to document lymphocytic infiltrates around blood vessels, such infiltrates may be only a small part of an entire disease process. Being careful "not to let the tail wag the dog," we must base our diagnosis of disease on the total clinical picture.

PRIMARY AND SECONDARY SJOGREN'S SYNDROME

Sjögren's syndrome may exist with other autoimmune disorders, for example, rheumatoid arthritis, systemic lupus erythematosus, and scleroderma. When a patient with dry eyes and/or dry mouth has one of these disorders, each of which has well accepted diagnostic criteria, the dryness conditions are termed *secondary Sjögren's syndrome.*

Other patients may have dry eyes and dry mouth along with symptoms of autoimmune disease, such as fatigue, fever, muscle aches, and joint pains, as well as characteristic laboratory abnormalities, such as elevated autoantibody levels in the bloodstream. If these clinical features do not fulfill criteria for any of the associated autoimmune diseases, these patients are termed *primary Sjögren's syndrome.*

The causes of primary SS may differ from the causes responsible for certain types of secondary SS. Individuals with primary SS have a different susceptibility gene, called HLA-DR3, than those with secondary SS and rheumatoid arthritis, who have a gene called HLA-DR4. These patient groups also differ in the specific antibodies, termed SS-A/Ro and SS-B/La, in their bloodstreams. Therefore, it is likely that more than one cause of Sjögren's syndrome will eventually be discovered.

GENES AND ENVIRONMENT

Most researchers think that Sjögren's syndrome and other autoimmune diseases result from the interaction of specific genetic susceptibility genes with particular environmental agents, that is, things present in the person's surroundings. For example, a patient with genetic susceptible gene HLA-DR3 may have an unusual immune response after infection with a particular virus or bacteria. As a result of these two factors, genes and environment, the immune system is tricked into mounting an immune attack on a particular target organ, such as the salivary glands.

Rheumatic fever is a well known example of the immune system making this kind of identity mistake. During a streptococcal bacterial infection, usually a strep throat, the immune system mounts a strong attack against this bacteria. However, because part of the immune system mistakes the normal lining cells of the heart valve as foreign or as similar to a part of the bacteria, it attacks and damages normal heart tissue.

AN EPSTEIN-BARR LINK?

What environmental agents initiate this process in Sjögren's syndrome? No one is sure. Indirect evidence suggests that viruses may play a role. Research interest has concentrated on the Epstein-Barr virus (EBV), a member of the herpesvirus family, which includes herpes simplex virus-1, the cause of cold sores, and varicella zoster virus, the cause of chicken pox and shingles.

EBV infection is very common in the United States, affecting over 90% of the population by age 20. Initial EBV infection usually leads to a mild flulike illness, occasionally with mildly swollen parotid glands. In most cases, the EBV infection is self-limited, and clinical recovery is rapid. A minority of individuals develop more severe clinical symptoms of fatigue and swollen lymph glands, a condition known as infectious mononucleosis.

In virtually everyone infected with EBV, including those with no symptoms, the virus establishes a "site of latency" or dormancy within the salivary gland, where it remains during our lifetime. Periodically, this latent EBV may be reactivated, as indicated by the presence of EBV in the saliva of healthy individuals. This reactivation probably occurs with other immunologic imbalances, such as during other viral infections that temporarily weaken the immune mechanisms that control EBV infections. Since nearly all normal adult individuals harbor EBV, no one should worry about being a carrier.

Some researchers believe that chronic fatigue is related to a so-called chronic EBV syndrome, but the existence of chronic EBV as a clinical entity and the relationship of chronic fatigue to the EBV virus remain highly controversial. Sjögren's syndrome is definitely not the same thing as chronic fatigue or chronic EBV.

A THEORY OF HOW SJOGREN'S SYNDROME DEVELOPS

Figure 1 depicts a model of Sjögren's syndrome. The first step in the development of the disorder, theoretically described as an extrinsic injury, refers to the salivary gland damage induced by some environmental agent. Although EBV is one potential candidate, no one has proved that this virus is the responsible agent.

Next, lymphocytes from the bloodstream migrate into the damaged salivary gland to help fight potential foreign invaders, such as viruses and bacteria. These lymphocytes can be divided into at least four groups:

(1) *B-cells*—produce antibodies after they receive particular signals from other lymphocytes;

(2) *T-helper cells*—provide the necessary signal for the B-cells;

(3) *T-killer cells*—recognize and destroy virus-infected cells;

(4) *T-suppressor cells*—decrease B-cell activity and T-killer cell production.

The infected salivary glands are damaged or cells are killed, either by the viral infection or by the lymphocytes, which attack the infected cell. As a result of cell death, substances within the salivary gland are released. Normally, the immune system ignores these "self substances." However, in SS patients, the self substances are mistakenly identified as "foreign" by the lymphocytes. Antibodies that are produced against self substances are called *autoantibodies,* and the substance itself is called an *autoantigen.*

For example, the B-cells produce autoantibodies that react with the nucleus of noninfected cells, the so-called *antinuclear antibodies* (ANAs) that we test for in SS patients. Of particular importance, antibodies are made against nuclear substances, called *Sjögren's syndrome-associated antigen A* (abbreviated SS-A) and *Sjögren's syndrome-associated antigen B* (SS-B), in a high proportion of SS patients. In some medical centers, the SS-A and SS-B autoantigens are referred to as the Ro and La autoantigens; however, the tests to detect SS-A/SS-B and Ro/La are identical. Thus, the results of these tests are interchangeable.

In addition to antinuclear antibodies, the B-cells also make an

autoantibody called *rheumatoid factor* (RF). This latter autoantibody received its name, because it was originally detected in the
blood of patients with rheumatoid arthritis. However, RF is also
present in SS patients who do not have rheumatoid arthritis and
serves as a useful marker of disease activity.

As a result of these lymphocyte responses, further damage to
the salivary gland may occur, stimulating a vicious cycle, wherein
more lymphocytes are attracted to the affected salivary gland. A
similar process occurs in the lacrimal and other moisture-secreting
glands. The process may continue until the glands are damaged so
much that clinical symptoms of dryness develop.

Defects involving T-suppresor cells may play a role, since
these cells are failing to regulate adequately the B-cells and T-
helper cells.

How do genetic factors contribute to this model? The ability
of T-cells and B-cells to respond to foreign or self substances is
governed by a group of genes called *human lymphocyte antigens*
(HLA). These HLA genes were first recognized during attempts to
transplant skin and other organs between different individuals. If
two individuals have identical HLA genes, transplantation can be
more easily achieved; if two individuals have different HLA genes,
the grafted tissue will be rejected rapidly by the recipient's lymphocytes.

From detailed studies of transplantation, it is known that at
least four different HLA genes (termed HLA-A, HLA-B, HLA-C,
and HLA-D) are involved. Of particular importance, the HLA-D
gene has been closely associated with Sjögren's syndrome, as well
as with other autoimmune diseases. There are at least 15 different
known HLA-D genes (HLA-D1, HLA-D2, HLA-D3, HLA-D4,
etc.), and each person has two different HLA-D genes, one inherited from each parent.

Individuals with HLA-D3 are at high risk for developing SS,
and individuals with HLA-D4 are at high risk for developing rheumatoid arthritis. In individuals with certain HLA-D genes, it is
likely that there is an increased chance that the immune system
may mistakenly attack self-antigens, particularly after a viral in-

fection. In other words, when the immune system of an individual with HLA-D3 encounters a particular virus in the salivary gland, there is an increased chance that it will mistakenly mount an incorrect attack on self tissues, leading to SS.

This hypothetical model of autoimmune disease is currently being investigated in many different laboratories to more precisely define the role of HLA-D genes and environmental agents.

Further studies on the genetic and environmental factors responsible for Sjögren's syndrome will allow earlier diagnosis and development of a specific cure, rather than our current symptomatic treatment.

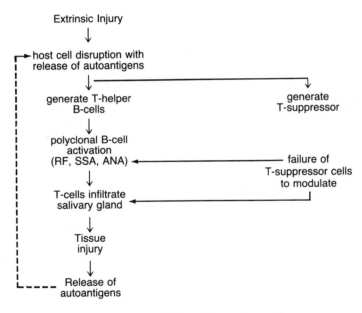

Figure 1.   Model for Sjögren's syndrome.

3

The Medical Workup

Steven Carsons, M.D.

Because individuals with Sjögren's syndrome (SS) have a variety of major symptoms and complaints, initially they may consult more than one specialist. They may go to an ophthalmologist for their eye problems; an otolaryngologist (physician specializing in ear, nose, and throat disorders) for their oral symptoms; and a dentist for problems with their teeth and salivary glands. These are the specialists who often diagnose SS.

Once diagnosed, Sjögren's syndrome patients will probably be referred to an internist with a special interest in SS for a thorough evaluation. Rheumatologists and clinical immunologists are specialists with the most experience in treating SS patients.

MEDICAL EVALUATION

The physician evaluating you for Sjögren's syndrome has four aims. First, he assesses your general health status. Second, he determines whether you are one of the 50% of SS patients who has an associated connective tissue (joint, skin, muscle) disorder, such as rheumatoid arthritis or systemic lupus erythematosus. Third, he searches for other autoimmune organ system disorders that may be associated with SS, such as thyroid disease. Finally, he ascertains your baseline immunologic status.

The most important technique the physician utilizes is a *comprehensive history,* the patient's verbal account of the symptoms and signs that prompted the visit to the doctor.

Next, the physician may ask a *series of questions* that do not immediately appear to be directly related to Sjögren's syndrome. However, these questions are used to probe for subtle signs that may point to an associated connective tissue or immune disorder. Typically, he may ask about joint aches, skin rashes, numbness of an extremity, or bruising and bleeding disorders.

The physician will inquire about the health of your family, particularly about family members who may have autoimmune or connective tissue disorders.

You will also be asked questions concerning habits, for example, smoking, alcohol consumption, and use of medications, both those prescribed by other physicians and "over-the-counter" (OTC) or self-prescribed items. Although these questions may seem irrelevant, each detail is important. Common antihistamines in OTC allergy or cold formulations, for instance, may greatly increase dryness. The same is true of diuretics (water pills) and many other classes of medications.

This discussion between physician and patient takes about 30 minutes, sometimes longer.

Next, the physician will perform a *general physical examination,* including careful inspection of the eyes, mouth, and the glands of the face and neck. The skin, joints, and scalp will be examined, as well as the heart, lungs, abdomen, and extremities.

After completing the physical examination, the doctor will order routine *blood tests* to check the blood count, liver and kidney function, and blood sugar level. He will test the erythrocyte sedimentation rate and perform several immunologic tests, described later in this chapter.

Because some patients with Sjögren's syndrome may have inflamed kidneys, a *urinalysis* is important. Similarly, the physician will want to see a *chest x-ray* to check the lungs for subtle signs of inflammation.

Following this comprehensive evaluation, the doctor will either wish to confer with other members of the team who have participated in your care or review records from other physicians.

After reviewing all available records, the doctor will address the question of whether or not you actually have Sjögren's syndrome. He will then consider whether any additional diagnostic tests are required to confirm the diagnosis.

ADDITIONAL DIAGNOSTIC TESTS

If an ophthalmologist has not already performed the *Schirmer test* (see illustration on page xxviii), your physician will now perform this simple screening examination. First, he will place a filter paper strip in the lower eyelid for a few minutes. He can easily measure the degree of wetting with a ruler. This is concrete, measurable evidence that the eyes are dry.

As noted in other chapters, dry eyes and dry mouth, known as the sicca complex or dryness complex, do not constitute a diagnosis of Sjögren's syndrome. Dryness may be caused by many other factors, among which are allergy, climate, medications, and aging.

Another eye test, usually performed by an ophthalmologist, is called the *slit lamp examination*. This test tells the physician whether there is an accompanying inflammation in the external eye structures, such as the cornea.

When the eyes are dry and chronically inflamed, the doctor will diagnose keratoconjuctivitis sicca (KCS). KCS alone does not mean that you have Sjögren's syndrome. However, if you have KCS and swollen salivary glands and/or a connective tissue disease, there is a high probability that you have Sjögren's syndrome.

The physician may evaluate salivary gland function. This is usually done simply by *careful inspection of the mouth*. In some instances, after stimulating saliva flow with a sour or acid substance, the doctor will collect and *measure the saliva*.

The salivary glands may be scanned with radioactive isotopes. After injecting *radioisotopes* into the bloodstream, x-rays of normal salivary glands show an uptake of the radioisotope. Individuals with Sjögren's syndrome, however, have a patchy and diminished uptake. Results of the scans generally correlate with the degree of salivary flow.

For detailed evaluation of the salivary glands, the doctor may order x-ray procedures, but these are not often used in routine clinical practice.

In one x-ray test, called *sialography,* a dye is injected into the salivary duct opening in the cheek, so that the entire ductal pattern can be seen. In Sjögren's syndrome, chronic inflammation causes an abnormal pattern. Although this is a useful test when a stone blocking a duct is suspected of causing salivary symptoms, sialography is usually not necessary to diagnose SS. The procedure is uncomfortable and sometimes makes symptoms worse. It is usually not performed on SS patients.

IMMUNOLOGICAL TESTS

Over the past several years, the discovery of many unique antibodies in the blood of Sjögren's syndrome patients has been helpful in making a diagnosis of SS.

The physician usually performs several *immunological tests* during his evaluation. None of these tests are diagnostic in and of themselves, but are very helpful when they are evaluated in conjunction with the clinical examination. Depending on the exact number of tests in an individual case, the cost ranges from $50 to $150.

Once immunological tests have been obtained during the initial evaluation, generally they are not repeated often. The following short glossary of currently used tests will help one understand how the physician uses these tests to help distinguish Sjögren's syndrome from other disorders.

The *erythrocyte sedimentation rate* (ESR) is the simplest and most basic test routinely used to evaluate patients suspected of having an inflammatory or connective tissue disorder. The test simply measures how rapidly a column of blood settles. If the ESR is elevated, you may have Sjögren's syndrome, particularly if you have an associated connective tissue disease. If the ESR is normal, a systemic inflammatory disorder (one involving many areas of the body) is less likely.

The doctor will also measure *immunoglobulins* or gamma globulins, normal blood proteins that protect you from disease. In Sjögren's syndrome and connective tissue disorders, immuno-globulins are generally elevated. Some physicians repeat immuno-globulin tests to follow the activity of SS.

The physician will also want to know whether there are an-tibodies called *rheumatoid factor* (RF) in your blood. Although this test is generally used as a screening examination for rheuma-toid arthritis (RA), RF may be found in individuals with other connective tissue diseases, as well as in those with SS. Therefore, the finding of a positive RF in an SS patient does not necessarily mean you have rheumatoid arthritis.

The *antinuclear antibody* (ANA) test is used as a screening tool for systemic lupus erythematosus (SLE or lupus.) Just as the rheumatoid factor is not found exclusively in rheumatoid arthritis patients, so ANAs are not restricted to people with lupus. They may be positive in other connective tissue diseases, in Sjögren's syndrome, and even following the use of certain medications. Therefore, the sole finding of positive ANA in an SS patient does not mean an individual also has lupus, especially if there are no other signs and symptoms of lupus.

Recently, a group of antibodies, called *Sjögren's antibodies,* has been found relatively frequently in people with SS. As other authors have discussed in previous chapters, the two classes of Sjögren's antibodies, first discovered in the blood of people with SS, are called SS-A or Ro and SS-B or La.

SS-A/Ro antibodies occur in 60% to 70% of SS patients, but are also found in people with other rheumatic or connective tissue disorders. SS-B/La antibodies are found in approximately 40% of people with SS, more commonly in those who have primary Sjö-gren's syndrome, that is, those who have no accompanying con-nective tissue disease.

HOW THE PHYSICIAN DIAGNOSES
SJOGREN'S SYNDROME

Once the physician has obtained all of your test results, including the ophthalmological examination performed by the eye doctor and the oral exam performed by the ear, nose, and throat specialist and/or the dentist, he is in a position to make a diagnosis of Sjögren's syndrome.

Before making a definite diagnosis, the doctor may recommend one last test, a small *biopsy of the inner portion of the lip.* This usually can be performed on an outpatient basis, often in a dentist's chair. The findings, reviewed by a pathologist, may give the physician an index of the inflammation and immunologic activity in the salivary glands and indicate whether the patient has Sjögren's syndrome.

Once the diagnosis has been made, it is extremely important that the ophthalmologist and dentist, as well as the internist, remain involved in the SS patient's care. You will see primarily the physicians or dentists who specialize in the part of your body that is presenting a particular problem. If you are primarily troubled with chronic eye irritation and inflammation, for example, you will see the ophthalmologist regularly. If you are suffering from recurrent dental and oral problems, you will see the oral specialist.

If you develop new symptoms or do not feel well, the rheumatologist or immunologist will wish to do a re-evaluation, perhaps checking a few blood tests to determine whether the new problem is related to SS and whether you require additional treatment.

Like everyone else, Sjögren's syndrome patients may have minor illnesses, such as colds, urinary tract infections, sprains, and muscle strains, so new symptoms may not be associated with SS and may require only routine medical treatment.

Although Sjögren's syndrome is a chronic illness, nearly all patients can lead productive lives. Currently, most physicians specializing in SS prefer to treat their patients conservatively, using preparations to restore or stimulate moisture production locally.

Because of chronic and potentially serious side effects, potent immunomodulating drugs, such as cortisone, are not routinely used to treat dryness or local swelling. These drugs are reserved for instances of severe inflammation of vital organs.

Monitoring and treatment by an appropriate health care team will help the Sjögren's syndrome patient feel more comfortable and prevent avoidable complications.

Part II

Glandular
Involvement

4

Eyes

R. Linsy Farris, M.D.

Blurred vision, intolerance to bright light, grittiness, burning, itching, and foreign body sensation are among common symptoms of the dry eye.

Paradoxically, excessive tearing is also a sign that the eye is dry. If resting state tearing (the amount of tears present when the eyes are not being stimulated) is not enough to properly moisten the eye, the eye produces reflex tears. When resting state tears are increased, reflex tearing subsides. Reflex tears normally occur whenever the eye is irritated by a foreign body, a gust of wind, a blast of air from an air conditioner, or anything that dries the surface of the eye.

Dry eye patients often notice that their symptoms worsen as the day progresses. Malfunctioning lacrimal (tear) glands cannot keep up with normal evaporative losses. Evaporation exceeds the rate of tear production, and the integrity of the tear film deteriorates as the day progresses.

Because the tear film is essential to providing a smooth surface on the front of the eye, where light rays are focused, blurred vision is often one of the first signs of a dry eye. A dry, somewhat roughened surface causes light rays to scatter, resulting in blurred vision. This is somewhat like looking through a dirty windshield.

Blinking several times to increase the tears on the surface of the cornea (the transparent structure up front in the eye, the "watch crystal" of the eye) will improve vision. So will any measure that increases the amount of moisture on the front of the cornea.

Providing increased liquid by means of artificial tear solutions may provide relief, but will not cure a dry eye condition. Relief is temporary, because artificial tears hydrate the tear film, but evaporate or drain away easily, unless the natural tear film is present.

MEDICAL CARE IS IMPORTANT

If you have dry eye symptoms, you should have a complete examination by an ophthalmologist, a physician specializing in eye disorders. The ophthalmologist will diagnose your condition and determine whether there is any ulceration, infection, or other ocular problem, which, untreated, could endanger your vision.

Patients frequently must search to find an ophthalmologist who has an interest in the dry eye and the patience to provide continuing care for a condition for which a cure is not yet available.

Dry eye patients should be under the regular care of an ophthalmologist. They should have checkups at least every six months, possibly more frequently, depending on the severity of symptoms and the state of eye disease.

WHAT ARE THE COMPONENTS
OF NORMAL TEAR FILM?

Because the dry eye involves much more than inadequate tears, the diagnosis is not easy. An abnormal tear film may be caused by abnormalities in the composition of any of the three layers of the film itself, in the eyelids, or in the cornea.

The tear film is a three-layer structure (see illustration on page xxvi), made up of mucus and fatty substances, as well as water and proteins (essential chemical components of all cells). The higher concentration of mucus on the surface of the cornea is called the *mucin layer*. The middle, watery layer that makes up most of our tear film is the *aqueous layer*. The outer, thin layer of fatty substance derived from the eyelids is the *lipid layer*.

The tear film is as complex as the blood and other body secretions. Any one of its components may be affected by eye disorders or disease, disrupting the continuous, intact film of liquid on the surface of the cornea.

WHAT IS THE ROLE OF THE MUCIN LAYER?

Mucin glands are scattered in the conjunctiva (the mucous membrane covering the outside of the eyeball and lining of the lids). By continuously secreting mucin, these glands provide the mucin component of tear film. Without adequate mucin lubrication, dry spots quickly develop on the cornea, leading to localized areas of tear deficiency. This stimulates corneal nerve endings, provoking the symptoms of dry eye described earlier.

WHAT IS THE ROLE OF THE AQUEOUS LAYER?

The main and accessory lacrimal glands deliver watery secretions into an accessory tear duct that empties into the upper conjunctiva, beneath the outer portion of the eyelid, and into the nasolacrimal tear duct. These watery secretions contain a variety of proteins, including *lysozyme* and *lactoferrin,* two of the antibacterial substances in tears that protect the eye against infections.

WHAT IS THE ROLE OF THE LIPID LAYER?

The fatty secretions of the tear film rest in a thin layer on the outer surface of the eye, protecting the eye by retarding evaporation of the tears. These fatty secretions work somewhat like paraffin placed on a jar of jelly. Lipid deficiency leads to excessive evaporation, which in turn leads to decreased tear volume and a dry eye.

In some cases, the fatty substances or lipids may be excessive, contaminating the underlying aqueous and mucin layers and resulting in dry spot formation.

Normally, these three layers of tear film appear to maintain a balance, preventing evaporation and continuously lubricating the surface of the cornea with tears.

WHAT ARE THE ROLES OF THE EYELIDS AND CORNEAL SURFACE?

In addition to the components in the three tear film layers, distribution of tears by the eyelids is extremely important. This permits tears to moisten and smooth out the eye surface. The surface of the cornea must also be normal and intact, to serve as a good foundation or base for the tear film.

Changes in the normal motion of the eyelids, as a result of an activity such as staring, cause excessive drying of the corneal surface. Neurological conditions that prevent spontaneous blinking are likely to produce a dry eye due to excessive evaporation. The corneal surface may also suffer from degenerations or diseases, called dystrophies, which may produce areas that cannot be resurfaced and covered by the normal tear film.

DIAGNOSTIC TESTS

The manifestations of the dry eye are subtle and may not be evident to the physician as he examines the eyes. Several diagnostic tests help determine whether one has a dry eye condition.

Diagnostic tests of tear film abnormalities vary greatly in their sensitivity (ability to obtain true positive results in patients with a disease) and their specificity (ability to determine normal subjects free of disease). Very seldom do tests have both a high sensitivity and a high specificity.

When using a set of criteria to compare a group of normals and a group of dry eye patients, all diagnostic tests will have an overlap of values, that is, a grey zone. This may obscure the true value and accuracy of the test. As a result, diagnostic tests are used only as a guide. The diagnosis is made by considering history, symptoms, and examination for signs of dry eye, as well as by diagnostic tests.

In the final analysis, the diagnosis of dry eye is a judgment, which becomes more definite as experience with the patient continues, both before and after various therapies are instituted.

SLIT LAMP EXAMINATION

In testing for dry eye, it is particularly important to avoid any stimulation that would produce reflex tearing, thereby masking a dry eye condition. In the *slit lamp examination,* which provides magnification without direct illumination, the eye can be viewed in its resting state, and examination of the basal tear volume is possible.

A wedge of tears, called the inferior marginal tear strip, usually rests on the lower eyelid margin. Its size may be a guide to the total volume of tears. Excessive debris in the tear film may be apparent, as well as a more viscous-appearing tear film and low-grade inflammation of the conjunctiva.

SCHIRMER TEST

Perhaps one of the best known tests for tear function, the *Schirmer test* (see illustration on page xxviii), is easily performed, with or without an anesthetic drop in the eye prior to the test. The only requirements are small strips of filter paper. When performed without anesthesia, this test may be viewed as a stress test, because of the stimulation caused by the dry filter paper when it touches the eyelid and conjunctiva.

The amount of stimulation varies greatly in individuals, however, resulting in immediate, complete wetting in some, and only 4 mm. or less of wetting in others. Besides sensitivity variations in normal individuals, various factors, such as alertness or allergies, may produce a wide variation of readings in the Schirmer strip.

If one uses very low values for the cutoff, such as 3 mm. of wetting in five minutes, the specificity (detection of normal eyes) of the test will be very high. However, the sensitivity in detecting patients who have dry eyes will be low.

ROSE BENGAL STAINING TEST

In the *rose bengal staining test,* the physician instills a red vegetable dye on the surface of the eye, which stains cells that have degenerated due to dryness.

After the dye is placed on the eye surface and allowed to rinse over the surface of the eye, the sides and central portion of the exposed eye are scored on a 0-to-3 scale for intensity of staining. The three areas are added together. The cutoff for a dry eye is a minimum score of 3.5.

This test is very specific for eyes that have a dry eye condition, but is not a very sensitive test. It frequently provides "normal" values in mild types of dry eye, thus producing a false negative test.

LYSOZYME AND LACTOFERRIN TESTS

Dry eye patients have decreased *lysozyme,* an enzyme (type of protein). The lysozyme test measures the amount of lysozyme in tears. When compared with a group of normal patients, there is considerable overlap of values, so it is difficult to be sure to which group an individual patient belongs. Moreover, the test is difficult to perform and is not useful to individual patients.

Lactoferrin is a more stable antibacterial enzyme in tears, which can now be measured with a new, readily available radial immunodiffusion plate (Lactoplate). The consistently reliable readings obtained in normal patients indicate that this may be a good test for dry eye.

TEAR OSMOLARITY TEST

The *tear osmolarity test* measures the particle concentration in tear film. For proper functioning, body fluids normally contain a certain concentration of salt. Tear osmolarity is a measure of this concentration, which in dry eye patients is hypertonic (much higher than normal).

A tiny amount of tear fluid is drawn and specially prepared for analysis. Because the test was developed to measure resting tears and to avoid contamination by reflex tears, which are present in so many other tests for dry eye, tear osmolarity appears to be more sensitive and specific than any of the other tests.

Presently, tear osmolarity is available as a diagnostic test in only a few centers. Its advantage to other tests is more accuate, quantitative information about the degree of dryness in the eyes.

FLUORESCEIN STAINING

Fluorescein is a vegetable dye that indicates points on the surface cells of the cornea that have rubbed off because of dryness. The dye is supplied in a strip, which is moistened by touching the inside of the lower eyelid, before the strip is instilled into the tears.

BREAKUP TIME (BUT)

Fluorescein is also useful in staining tears to detect how well the cornea remains continuously covered with a tear film. Breakup time (BUT) tests how well the cornea remains moistened between blinks. After moistening a filter paper strip containing fluorescein with a nonpreserved saline solution, the fluorescein is instilled into the tears. Next, the patient blinks, then holds the eyes open for 10 seconds. When a dry spot appears on the cornea, the breakup time is determined. A value less than 10 seconds indicates a dry eye state. Hypofluorescence is sometimes observed while doing this test; this may be used as an additional clinical indicator of low tear volume and a dry eye.

HOW MUCH DO THESE TESTS COST?

The cost of these tests varies widely by locality and the physician's expertise. In many cases, the Schirmer test may be done merely as an addition to the regular eye examination. The tear osmolarity test, on the other hand, requires a technician and very precise electronic equipment. As a result, tear osmolarity is the most expensive test, requiring an additional fee.

FIRST SYMPTOMS OF DRY EYE

The dry eye can fluctuate considerably. Not only is the eye affected by abnormal tear composition, it is also sensitive to environmental agents, such as low humidity, dust, and smoke. Its small size and small tear volume make it sensitive to evaporation.

Fortunately, corneal nerve endings warn the individual when the eye is becoming dry. Only in certain neurological disorders, in which sensation and lid blinking are disturbed, would the eye be likely to become dry without an awareness. In addition to the sensation of dryness, redness of the eye is likely to develop, as well as blurred vision. One of these three symptoms is usually sufficient to warn the patient and lead to a visit to an ophthalmologist.

TREATMENTS FOR DRY EYE

Current treatments are numerous, ranging from artificial tear solutions to plugging of the lacrimal puncta, the entrance to the drainage system for tears.

ARTIFICIAL TEARS

Tear substitutes containing preservatives may become toxic, particularly if they are used more than six times a day. Artificial tear drops used more frequently may also rinse away the normal tears needed to re-establish a normal tear film. Preservative-free solutions are prone to bacterial contamination; thus they are frequently packaged in single dose vials. Preservative-free solutions should be kept cold and used over a period of not more than 24 to 36 hours.

Although many dry eye patients use ointments, particularly at bedtime, some patients feel that ointments dry out in the eye, increasing foreign body sensation, while others feel that ointments cause blurred vision on awakening.

Artificial tears primarily increase comfort. If the solution makes one more uncomfortable or burns, it is probably creating a toxic or sensitivity reaction. Another brand of artificial tears or a switch to a sterile, preservative-free solution should be attempted. (Tear substitutes are listed at the end of this chapter.)

THE LACRISERT

The *Lacrisert* is a small, chemical polymer rod that absorbs water and slowly dissolves, producing a film over normal tears. The film conserves tears by preventing evaporation. Unfortunately, a fair number of individuals have difficulty inserting the very small pellet beneath the lower eyelid. Many dry eye patients have an increased foreign body sensation after they insert the rod.

Artificial tears must be used with the Lacrisert to supplement it and help it dissolve. For those with mild to moderate dry eye conditions, Lacriserts often provide increased comfort.

MOISTURE CHAMBER EYEGLASSES

Moisture chamber eyeglasses are extremely helpful in conserving the small volume of tears in dry eye patients. Used in addition to tear substitutes, these custom-made eyeglasses also protect the eyes from exposure to air currents, such as air conditioning and wind gusts, and are helpful during a long automobile trip or during air travel.

(See Appendix B for a guide for opticians who wish to make moisture chamber eyeglasses for dry eye patients.)

PUNCTAL OCCLUSION

Punctal occlusion (closure of the tear ducts, to provide an increased volume of tears by decreasing drainage) is accomplished in several ways. Whatever method is used, the lower puncta are usually sealed first. Depending on subsequent improvement in symptoms, the upper puncta may be sealed later.

There are two types of punctal plugs, collagen and silicone. The collagen plug lasts only two to three weeks and is eventually absorbed. This can help both patient and physician evaluate the reaction to the plugs.

The silicone plug, on the other hand, is not absorbed, but it can be removed easily. This is important. If the patient's condition improves, and tears are once again produced in greater amounts, the plug will no longer be needed.

Just as connective tissue diseases vary, so a dry eye condition can vary in its severity. Fluctuation in tear production is not uncommon in patients who are believed to be in the early stages of Sjögren's syndrome.

As a last resort, the puncta can be closed surgically by electrocautery or by Argon laser. Surgical occlusion may or may not prove successful. It is extremely difficult to reverse.

VITAMIN A OINTMENT

Vitamin A ointment (Tretinoin) is now under investigation. Current studies indicate it may be helpful for patients with relatively rare, severe dry eye conditions. New studies to further evaluate the drug are underway.

COMMON PROBLEMS

After starting artificial tear therapy, many patients are disappointed. They may expect a complete cure or become tired of repeatedly instilling artificial tear drops to obtain relief. Like many skin conditions, the dry eye is frequently helped by medication, but hardly ever completely cured.

To become efficient and avoid drenching your face, instilling tear drops takes practice. Excessive drops on the lashes should be removed with a clean tissue or cotton pad, since rapid drying on the lid margin may lead to flakes, which can irritate the eye.

Tap water should never be instilled into the eye, because even the best city water supplies may contain bacteria. Any solution instilled into the eye must be sterile and, if free of preservatives, used no later than 36 hours after opening. Even sterile solutions should not be kept more than three months, once the bottles are opened.

Lid hygiene will make one more comfortable. Warm compresses soften dried secretions from the lid margin, which then can be removed with a dry Q-tip.

General body hygiene, with the use of shampoo and soap containing antibacterial compounds, is important to decrease the number of bacteria living on the skin. Bacteria gaining entrance to a dry eye with decreased local resistance may lead to bacterial infections. Rubbing the eyes with soiled tissues or dirty fingers is asking for trouble.

Having the eyes examined periodically by a medical doctor, following his advice, and properly using medications will prevent damage to vision and usually permit maximum comfort.

CATARACT SURGERY AND DRY EYE PATIENTS

Dry eye patients undergoing cataract surgery can expect a slightly greater degree of irritation and a longer period, up to 10 weeks, before complete visual recovery is obtained. Fortunately, a dry eye is superficial and usually does not interfere with wound healing. Continued treatment of the dry eye during the recovery period is sometimes necessary, in spite of increased stimulation of reflex tears afforded by the operative wound.

BLEPHARITIS

Blepharitis (inflammation of the eyelids) is a common cause of the dry eye. This frequently requires treatment, before the physician can accurately assess lacrimal gland function.

Blepharitis may arise from several factors, but appears related primarily to the secretions from the numerous meibomian glands in the eyelid, which release secretions through openings in the upper and lower lid margins. In blepharitis, the secretions appear excessive and seem to clog the openings on the lid margin, leading to reddened lid margins, crusts, granulations, small ulcers, styes, and chalazion (a small bump) on the eyelid margin.

Blepharitis causes constant and severe discomfort, not only because of the lid disease, but because of the accompanying dry eye, which apparently results from abnormalities in the lipid layer of tear film. Blepharitis may cause both an inadequate amount of lipid due to clogged glands, or to an excessive amount of lipid due to oversecretion or failure to remove secretions from the lids every day.

TREATMENT FOR BLEPHARITIS

Blepharitis is treated by applying warm compresses to the lids, using tap water and an ordinary bath cloth. By maintaining heat on the lids for five to 10 minutes, depending on the severity of the blepharitis, the lipid secretions of the lid are softened, so that they can be removed more easily from the lid and gland openings. After removing the warm compresses, firmly rub the lid margins behind the eye lashes with a tightly wound, cotton-tipped applicator. A magnifying makeup mirror will help to place the applicator correctly.

Some physicians recommend using baby shampoo or special soaps and pads to cleans the lids. Individuals should use what works best for them. One approach is to make the routine as simple as possible, since such chores, like brushing and flossing teeth after every meal, frequently are not done by those in a rush to do other things that seem more important.

The use of baby shampoo on the eyelid, however, particularly if one has trouble keeping the shampoo confined to the lid margin, risks getting it into the tear film, where it will interfere with tear film function.

Many patients with blepharitis question whether their condition will ever go away, or will they have to continue this manner of lid hygiene indefinitely. Since blepharitis is really more of a skin condition than a disease, the condition most likely will remain indefinitely to some degree, depending on many factors, such as perspiration and gland secretion.

Eye rubbing with unwashed fingers and inadequate removal of oils, makeup, and secretions will make blepharitis worse. Regular lid hygiene will not only make blepharitis better, by preventing inflammation and symptoms of dry eye, it will also prevent infections of the eyelids, such as styes and lid ulcerations.

Regular attention to cleaning the lid margins illustrates the adage, "An ounce of prevention is worth a pound of cure."

ACTIVITIES AND CONDITIONS THAT AGGRAVATE THE EYE

- Reading and study, prolonged work at a computer terminal, and concentration are activities that decrease the blink rate. Try blinking on purpose.
- Low humidity.
- Air conditioning.
- Air currents.
- Dust and fumes.
- Smoke.
- Excessive makeup, especially on the eyelid margin. Makeup is all right, as long as it is kept mainly on the tips of the eyelashes and the skin of the lid. If it is applied too close to the base of the eyelash, it tends to soften and run, allowing it to enter the tear film and result in more concentrated tears.
- Parasympatholytic drugs, drugs that make the mouth dry, such as tranquilizers, antihistamines, and others.

ARTIFICIAL TEAR PREPARATIONS (Demulcents)
Compounded by the Manufacturer

Major Component	Trade Name	Preservative
Gum cellulose	Celluvisc (1%)[1,2]	— (unit dose)
Hydroxyethylcellulose	Clerz	thimerosal + edetate disodium
	Lyteers	benzalkonium chloride + edetate disodium
	Teargard	thimerosal + edetate disodium
Hydroxypropylcellulose	Lacrisert*	benzalkonium chloride + edetate disodium
Hydroxypropyl methylcellulose	Isopto Alkaline	benzalkonium chloride
	Isopto Plain	benzalkonium chloride
	Isopto Tears	benzalkonium chloride
	Lacril	chlorobutanol
	Muro Tears	benzalkonium chloride + edetate disodium
	Tearisol	benzalkonium chloride + edate disodium
	Tears Naturale II[2]	Polyquad + edetate disodium
Methylcellulose	Methopto	benzalkonium chloride
	Methulose	benzalkonium chloride
	Murocel	methylparaben + propylparaben
	Visculose	benzalkonium chloride
Polyvinyl alcohol	Aqua Tears	benzalkonium chloride + edetate sodium
	Liquifilm Tears	chlorobutanol
	Liquifilm Forte	thimerosal + edate disodium
	Tears Plus	chlorobutanol
Polyvinyl alcohol and cellulose ester	aqua-FLOW	benzalkonium chloride + edetate disodium
	Neo-Tears	thimerosal + edetate disodium
Polyvinyl alcohol and povidone	Refresh	— (unit dose)
Other Polymeric Systems	Adapettes	thimerosal + edetate disodium
	Adsorbotear	thimerosal + edetate disodium
	Comfort Drops	benzalkonium chloride + edetate disodium
	Dual Wet	benzalkonium chloride + edetate disodium
	Hypo Tears	benzalkonium chloride + edetate disodium
	Tears Naturale	benzalkonium chloride + edetate disodium

Compounded by a Registered Pharmacist

Gum cellulose, preservative-free (.3%, .625%, .95%, 1.25%)*[2]
Healon tears*[2]
Methylcellulose (0.5%), preservative free*[2]

OCULAR EMOLLIENTS

Trade Name	Composition
Akwa-Tears (Akorn)	Petrolatum, liquid lanolin, mineral oil.
Duolube (Muro)	Sterile ointment containing white petrolatum and mineral oil.
Duratears Naturale (Alcon)[2]	Preservative-free sterile ointment with white petrolatum, liquid lanolin, and mineral oil.
Hypo Tears (Cooper Vision)	Sterile ointment containing white petrolatum and light mineral oil.
Lacri-lube S.O.P. (Allergan)	Sterile ointment with 42.5% mineral oil, 55% white petrolatum, lanolin, and chlorobutanol.
Refresh P.M. (Allergan)[2]	Preservative-free sterile ointment containing white petrolatum 55%, mineral oil 41.5%, petrolatum and lanolin alcohol 2%.

*Prescription medication; all other preparations are nonprescription.

1. New product scheduled to be available for purchase in Spring of 1989.

2. Except for the seven products marked "2", the above material is adapted from tables in the 1988 edition of the *PDR FOR OPHTHALMOLOGY.*

5

Mouth

Troy E. Daniels, D.D.S., M.S.
Irwin D. Mandel, D.D.S.
James J. Sciubba, D.M.D., Ph.D.

Saliva is one of our natural resources. Too often the bounty of a natural resource is not appreciated until there is a shortage.

Patients with Sjögren's syndrome (SS) have different amounts of reduction in their saliva flow. However, in all but the most severe patients, there is some increase in this flow following stimulation with taste or chewing. In many patients, however, there is little saliva flow without stimulation. Therefore, at rest, the SS patient's mouth may be completely dry.

People with SS may also have other diseases that require the long-term use of medication for treatment. Many of these medications can reduce salivary flow as a side effect, thus compounding the problem of the SS patient. Since saliva is a complex fluid, containing a variety of components and serving many physiologic needs, a marked shortage of this fluid can produce discomfort; impair oral function in chewing, swallowing, and speaking; and lead to damage to the teeth and oral mucous membranes.

Saliva is produced by three pairs of major salivary glands: the *parotid* glands, located in front of the ears; the *submandibular* glands, located below the lower jaw; and the *sublingual* glands, located in the floor of the mouth, under the tongue. These major glands produce about 95% of the saliva. The rest comes from numerous, pinhead-size, minor salivary glands, located in many areas of the mouth, just beneath the surface. The number of these minor glands is especially high in the areas of the lips and palate. In SS, both the major and minor glands are affected. Patients have very different levels of salivary dysfunction and overall intensity of symptoms.

SPECIFIC FUNCTIONS OF SALIVA

A brief discussion of the specific functions of saliva will help in understanding how and why oral problems occur when there is not enough saliva.

Contrary to common belief, the main function of saliva is not the digestion of starches. Saliva does indeed contain a large amount of the enzyme amylase, which digests starch, but the pancreas also produces a great deal of amylase. Saliva as a source of amylase is not critical.

The contribution of the salivary secretions to ingestion and digestion of food is mainly preparative and gastronomic. The mucin (mucouslike component) in saliva covers the food bolus and helps move it along the chewing and swallowing surfaces. Other components of saliva provide the appropriate environment for the taste buds to function.

Since we are not eating most of the time, the salivary glands are not responding to taste or chewing stimuli. Yet they are secreting a small amount of fluid, helping to maintain the structure of the teeth and mucous membranes of the mouth and throat. The combined saliva from the major and minor salivary glands contains a variety of salts, proteins, carbohydrates, and lipids (fats), which give it considerable protective properties.

Saliva has five major protective functions:

(1) *Coating and lubrication of the mucous membranes.* In addition to covering the food bolus, mucin sticks to and coats all the tissues of the mouth. This material produces the smooth sensation one normally feels when one runs the tongue over the lips, teeth, and gums. The mucin coating serves as a natural barrier to

irritating components in food and beverages, as well as to toxic products generated by bacteria in the mouth and to the dehydrating effect of mouth breathing. This coating on the teeth and soft tissues also allows for ready passage of the food bolus and enables the teeth to glide smoothly over each other during chewing.

(2) *Mechanical cleansing.* The flow of saliva and the muscle activity of the lips and tongue remove most food remnants and large numbers of potentially harmful bacteria from the teeth and soft tissues. The maximal effect is during eating, when the combination of taste and chewing stimulation produces the maximal flow of saliva. This clearance mechanism is similar to tearing and blinking in the eye, blowing the nose, and coughing to clear the lungs.

(3) *Maintenance of neutrality.* Saliva contains components that buffer and neutralize acidic and basic (alkaline) foods and beverages, helping to keep the oral cavity at a neutral level (pH of 7.0). If the oral environment is too acidic or too basic, the tissues can become irritated. The saliva also affects acid formation in the bacterial plaques that form on tooth surfaces. These bacterial plaques can convert the various kinds of sugar in the diet into acids that initiate tooth decay. A normal salivary flow provides a continuous source of buffering substances that flow into the bacterial plaques, neutralizing the acids as they are formed.

(4) *Maintenance of tooth structure.* Teeth are made up of a crystalline substance, composed mainly of calcium and phosphate in a special configuration (hydroxyapatite). To prevent dissolution of these crystals, normal saliva contains an appropriate concentration of calcium and phosphate salts, kept in balance by specialized proteins. In the absence or severe reduction of saliva, this equilibrium between the calcium and phosphate in the tooth and in the saliva is disturbed, and teeth are more susceptible to decay and direct erosion by acid foods and beverages. The mucin coatings on the teeth, described above, are also protective against erosion, abrasion, or abnormal physical wear.

(5) *Antibacterial activity.* In addition to physically removing bacteria, saliva can affect bacteria in other ways. Coating of bac-

teria by mucin and other salivary proteins causes clumping of the bacteria, so they cannot stick to teeth or soft tissues and are swallowed. A special antibody in saliva, called secretory IgA, can also coat oral bacteria, preventing their attachment to teeth or soft tissues. A group of salivary proteins (lysozyme, lactoferrin, and salivary peroxidase), working in conjunction with other components of saliva, can have an immediate effect on oral bacteria, interfering with their ability to multiply or killing them directly.

DIAGNOSIS OF ORAL PROBLEMS IN SJOGREN'S SYNDROME

Early diagnosis of Sjögren's syndrome needs to be made, so damage to teeth and eyes can be prevented. But SS must be carefully diagnosed to distinguish between the various causes of symptoms of dry eyes and dry mouth. Because SS is chronic in all patients and progressive in some, assigning the diagnosis inappropriately can cause a patient years of unnecessary concern about his or her health. No one test will establish the presence of SS. Therefore, each component (salivary, ocular, and systemic) is diagnosed separately. Two out of these three components must be established by reliable, objective diagnostic criteria for SS to be confirmed.

Although dry mouth is a part of most definitions of Sjögren's syndrome and is certainly an important problem for most patients, it is an unsatisfactory basis on which to diagnose the salivary component of SS. Symptoms of dry mouth are interpreted differently by the patients experiencing them, and dry mouth can be caused by a variety of conditions in addition to SS. The most common cause of dry mouth symptoms is the effect of many prescription medications, as noted above.

The various means of assessing salivary glands include: measuring the amount of saliva, x-ray examination of the glands, nuclear medicine examination, measuring components of saliva, and salivary gland biopsy. All these methods have a role in the diagnosis of various salivary gland diseases, but they are not equally helpful in diagnosing the salivary component of SS.

Measuring the amount of saliva. Salivary flow rates can be measured for whole saliva (from all the glands) or for parotid or submandibular gland secretions separately, either unstimulated or stimulated by taste or chewing. Unstimulated whole salivary flow rates measure a patient's basal or resting salivary secretion. These rates, which are reduced in SS, most closely reflect a patient's symptoms of dry mouth. But they are also reduced by the side effects of many commonly prescribed drugs and by diseases other than SS.

Separate flow rates from parotid or submandibular glands, measured with taste or chewing stimulation, give an estimate of the amount of saliva the gland can secrete. However, these rates are proportional to the size of the gland, which varies greatly among individuals. Standardized measurements of stimulated salivary flow are useful in determining a person's salivary gland function and offer a noninvasive way to follow the course of a chronic disease such as SS. However, they are too variable and nonspecific (caused by diseases other than SS) to serve as a diagnostic test for SS.

X-ray examination. Sialography is a method for examining changes in the duct system of the major salivary glands. Liquid contrast medium (a substance visible by x-ray) is injected slowly into the salivary gland though its duct opening in the mouth. This has been used to examine patients with SS, but has important disadvantages: the changes revealed by this test are not specific to SS; some of the x-ray contrast media used in this technique can cause unacceptable side effects; and safer x-ray contrast media are less effective in detecting changes in the ducts.

Nuclear medicine examination. Sequential salivary scintigraphy is a diagnostic technique involving injection of a tiny quantity of radioactive material into a vein. The radioactive material soon localizes in the major salivary glands, and is detectable by examination of the head and neck with a special and very sensitive camera that can locate the radioactive material. This can be used to assess the function of the major salivary glands simultaneously.

In SS patients, the rate that the radioactive material is taken up by the glands and the rate that radioactive saliva appears in the mouth are delayed or absent. Salivary scintigraphic findings correlate with stimulated parotid flow rate measurements, but these findings are not diagnostically specific for SS.

Measuring salivary components. Measuring the amount of various chemical or immunological constituents in saliva is called sialochemistry. In several studies with SS patients, these measurements have shown some promising results, promoting better understanding of the salivary component of this disease. At the moment, none of these measurements are yet sufficiently specific to serve as diagnostic tests.

Salivary gland biopsy. Labial salivary gland biopsy (microscopically examining minor salivary glands from the inside of the lower lip) offers the most disease-specific way to diagnose the salivary component of SS. The microscope reveals the characteristic disease process of SS, which is a distinctive pattern of infiltration of the affected glands by lymphocytes (a type of white blood cell). These infiltrates are similar to those seen in any of the organs affected by SS, including the salivary glands, lacrimal (tear) glands, liver, kidney, or lungs. These infiltrates cause the affected organs to function abnormally, producing such symptoms as dry mouth or dry eyes.

Because SS is a systemic disease, it affects both major and minor salivary glands. Biopsy of minor glands avoids the need to biopsy a major gland, usually the parotid, which can produce facial scarring, nerve damage, and salivary fistula formation (abnormal drainage of saliva through the skin of the face). Recent studies have described safer ways to biopsy the parotid gland, but these specimens are less satisfactory for diagnosing the salivary component of SS than labial (lip) glands, expecially for patients with early or mild disease.

A labial salivary gland biopsy involves removal of several pinhead-size minor glands under local anesthesia. Performed as an outpatient procedure, the salivary gland biopsy can reveal the characteristic infiltration pattern of SS. The biopsy will not make the patient's dry mouth worse. In the absence of SS, the biopsy may reveal other causes of a patient's dry mouth.

CLINICAL FEATURES

Symptoms (changes patients feel). The principal oral symptom of SS is dryness, often called xerostomia. However, not all patients describe their problem this way. Some may mention difficulty in swallowing food, problems in wearing complete dentures, changes in the sense of taste, burning symptoms in the mouth, or inability to eat dry foods. These symptoms usually have a very gradual onset. In some patients, the severity of these symptoms may fluctuate slowly over periods of weeks or months.

Signs (changes that can be seen or measured). The parotid or the submandibular glands in SS may show various degrees of firm enlargement, usually without tenderness. About one-third of patients with SS will develop this enlargement in their major salivary glands at some time, but most SS patients will not have this problem. Many SS patients with major salivary gland enlargement report that it occurs in episodes lasting for many weeks or months, while other patients have chronic enlargement with slow changes in size. The swelling may begin on one side, but affects both sides eventually.

Angular cheilitis (sores at the angles of the lips) is a common feature of those patients who have oral candidiasis (overgrowth inside the mouth of a common oral yeast called *Candida*). This overgrowth occurs as a result of changes in the saliva of many, but not all patients with SS.

The intraoral (inside the mouth) signs of patients with SS are similar in appearance to those in patients with chronic xerostomia of any cause. These include: (1) dry, sticky oral mucosal surfaces; (2) dental caries (decay), primarily affecting the teeth at the gum line or on the incisal (cutting) edges of the front teeth; (3) cloudy saliva or no saliva expressible from the parotid or submandibular ducts; (4) smooth or cobblestone appearance of the tongue, with or without fissures; and (5) areas of redness on the roof of the mouth, inside the cheeks, under dentures, or on the tongue. Signs (4) and (5) are usually associated with the symptom of burning.

Tooth decay. One of the earliest and most common oral problems in patients with SS is an increase in tooth decay. The marked reduction in saliva volume, along with the associated loss of its protective and antibacterial properties, result in an increased retention of bacterial plaque and food debris around the teeth, especially at the gum line. Not only is there more plaque, but the nature of the plaque changes. With a reduction in salivary flow, the saliva becomes acidic. A less protective, more acidic saliva causes a change in the balance of the various bacterial organisms that make up plaque. Organisms that live well in such an environment thrive at the expense of their neighbors. *Streptococcus mutans,* the bacteria with the greatest potential for producing decay, rapidly increases in number.

As if this shift were not enough, when many people first experience the dry mouth feeling, they often use candies, mints, or gum to stimulate the flow of saliva. Sugar provides bacteria in the plaque with an ideal environment for producing destructive acids on the tooth surfaces. Use of sugar-containing agents leads rapidly to decay. Therefore, nonsucrose sweeteners, such as sorbitol, mannitol, xylitol, or Nutrasweet should be used.

In people with dry mouth, the most vulnerable part of the tooth is at the gum line. In older individuals who have recession of the gums, the exposed cementum or dentin can be attacked very rapidly, resulting in root caries. Tooth enamel is also susceptible, especially at the margins of old fillings, where there may be chips, breaks, and roughness. "My fillings are falling out" is a common complaint. The junctions of tooth surfaces with gold, plastic, or porcelain crowns (caps) are also very vulnerable to tooth decay.

In the severely dry mouth, however, all surfaces are at at risk, even those not usually susceptible to decay, such as the edges of the incisor teeth.

Tooth erosion and abrasion. In addition to tooth decay, tooth substance can be lost by the direct attack of acids contained in food, beverages, and confections, as well as by abrasion due to physical forces.

Excessive use of citrus fruits or frequent use of sour candies should be avoided. Moderation is the key. Soft drinks, which are all very acidic, should be used with a straw to bypass the teeth. Soft drinks should not contain sucrose. The teeth should be brushed with a soft toothbrush, using moderate pressure. Overly abrasive toothpastes (those designed for smokers or people with heavy tooth stains) should be avoided.

Gingivitis and periodontitis. The increased retention of plaque on the teeth can result in gingivitis (inflammation of the gums). This is controllable with good oral hygiene. However, there is no evidence that the more serious form of periodontal disease, periodontitis (inflammation of the tissues surrounding and supporting the teeth), is increased in patients with dry mouth. The changes occurring in the balance between different types of bacteria in the mouth apparently do not result in an increase of the bacteria that cause periodontal disease. In people with existing periodontitis, special attention has to be given to oral hygiene, because periodontal pockets, spaces between the gums and the teeth, are vulnerable to decay.

Soft tissues. In xerostomia, the oral soft tissues become very dry, smooth, and shiny. They have a parched appearance and are often sticky or tacky when touched with fingers or instruments. The appearance of the tongue may range from slight reddening and mild fissuring to severe deep fissures. These changes are usually caused by the candidiasis described below. Patients wearing complete dentures have special difficulties. The lack of a lubricating salivary film may allow the tongue to stick to the dentures, especially the lower, causing it to move and leading to sore spots and ulcerations.

Yeast overgrowth. It is not uncommon to find soft white patches or streaks on the tongue, cheeks, or palate, often accompanied by burning and tenderness, especially under a complete denture. This condition is due to an overgrowth of the yeast *Candida,* an organism usually present in very small numbers in the mouth. With reduction in salivary flow and marked changes in the chemical and physical nature of the oral environment, yeasts can grow in great numbers at the expense of their neighbors. Specific antifungal drugs are required to treat this. Even with effective initial treatment, this overgrowth often recurs and must be re-treated.

Miscellaneous problems. In some patients, a variety of other oral disturbances can occur, including difficulties in swallowing, oral malodor, and changes in the sense of taste. The taste problems range from intolerance to spicy foods and strong flavors to difficulty in recognizing the normal taste characteristics of specific foods. These problems may improve with adequate treatment of oral candidiasis. The swallowing difficulty arises from the lack of an adequate mucin coating on the food bolus and oral mucosa, which interferes with the ability of the food to move smoothly from the back of the mouth to the esophagus. Constant sipping of water during meals is necessary. Oral malodor can arise from retention of food remnants in the mouth and overgrowth of certain bacteria, making scrupulous oral hygiene essential.

TREATING DRY MOUTH

While SS is not curable, it is certainly manageable to the extent of reducing a patient's symptoms and preventing irreversible damage to the teeth and eyes. Managing the salivary component of SS includes: treating and preventing dental caries, reducing oral mucosal symptoms by treating and retreating oral candidiasis, stimulating remaining salivary glands to produce more saliva, and using saliva substitutes.

Dental caries. The cause of dental decay from xerostomia has been discussed. Decay usually attacks the teeth next to the gingiva (gums) and at the junctions of dental fillings or crowns, even those located under the gingiva. Since decay in these areas can be very difficult to treat and the problems of dry mouth may be continuous, preventing decay is an important aspect of oral treatment for all SS patients with remaining teeth. Although not everything is known about the cause of this type of decay, it is clear that daily use of topical fluoride preparations can significantly reduce or eliminate the dental decay, even in patients with severe dry mouth.

Methods of preventing new and recurrent dental caries in patients with SS need to be individualized by their dentists, according to the patient's dental status and severity of xerostomia. A reasonable level of prevention for a patient who has continuous dry mouth, but some remaining salivary function, should include: (1) daily fluoride mouth rinsing for one to two minutes before going to bed, without rinsing with water afterwards; (2) discontinuing all sugar-containing foods or beverages between meals; (3) careful daily removal of plaque deposits from the teeth; and (4) regular dental supervision and care.

Patients with more severe xerostomia may require longer application of fluoride and the use of custom-fitted plastic trays made by their dentist that fit over their teeth and carry a fluoride gel. Fluoride tablets and fluoridated water supplies, which help prevent tooth decay in children, are of no help to adults, because both methods work by providing fluoride internally to teeth that are forming. Fully formed adult teeth cannot use this form of fluoride.

Remineralizing solutions. Prior to actual cavity formation, there is a loss of calcium and phosphate from the tooth surface and below. These minerals of the tooth enamel are deposited on a scaffold or matrix. In the earliest phases of cavity formation, the matrix remains behind as the mineral is lost. The daily use of remineralizing solutions as a rinse helps the matrix once again hold the minerals previously lost due to acid buildup in the dry mouth. These solutions must be mixed just prior to rinsing from two separate "A" and "B" components: one rich in calcium salts and the other rich in phosphate salts. In combination with fluoride, this adjunct in the dry mouth helps prolong a healthy dental status.

Oral candidiasis. As described above, many of the changes occurring on the oral mucous membranes are caused by overgrowth of a common yeast called *Candida,* which is not harmful normally. This happens in about one-third of patients with SS as a result of their dry mouth and other unknown factors.

Antifungal drugs applied topically or on the surface of the mouth for periods of several weeks to several months can eliminate the yeast overgrowth (called atrophic or erythematous oral candidiasis) and the changes it causes in the mucosa, allowing the oral mucosa to return to normal. (Atrophic refers to a thinning of the surface of the mucosa, causing burning symptoms and predisposing to discomfort and ulcers.) This treatment is important, because it improves the oral comfort of most patients, even though the dryness continues. Many antifungal drugs are available by prescription, but all are not equally effective and a number of them contain sugar, which can increase the risk of dental decay, if used chronically.

Patients who wear removable dentures need to remove their dentures and apply the antifungal medicine directly in the mouth. The dentures themselves also need to be treated to eliminate the yeast. Additionally, individuals wearing partial or complete dentures are encouraged to remove them at bedtime and, after thoroughly cleansing them, to soak them overnight in a suitable solution prescribed by their dentist. This will also help eliminate the yeast problem.

The diagnosis and management of oral candidiasis is usually best carried out by the patient's dentist. Even after successful treatment, however, many patients will have the problem recur, so they should be routinely re-examined and may require chronic treatment.

Salivary stimulation. Attempts to relieve the symptoms of oral dryness and restore salivary function have taken two approaches: stimulation of the salivary glands to secrete more saliva and use of saliva substitutes. Saliva can be stimulated through the sense of taste or by chewing. Regular use of sugarless, hard candies or sugarless chewing gum produces this kind of stimulation, but it occurs only while the stimulus is applied.

More recently, an electronic device to stimulate salivary flow has become available. Tests of its effectiveness show that, while in use, it can increase salivary flow in some patients with SS, but only in those with some residual salivary function. Patients with very low or no salivary flow did not respond.

The drug pilocarpine has been shown to increase saliva production in patients with the severe xerostomia following radiation therapy to the head and neck. Patients with SS may also find it helpful, but prospective studies have not yet been done. A single oral dose of pilocarpine can give up to two hours of stimulation. However, side effects of sweating or stomach cramping may be encountered with this drug. Pilocarpine cannot be used in patients with a history of gastrointestinal ulcer and should be used with caution in patients with high blood pressure or other cardiovascular diseases. Effects of its long-term use are unknown.

Other drugs have been used to stimulate salivary and tear production in patients with Sjögren's syndrome. Short-term use of the drug anetholetrithione, called Sulfarlem in Europe and Sialor in Canada, is generally able to stimulate salivary flow in patients with mild xerostomia from SS, but not in patients with severe dry mouth. It cannot be used in patients with chronic liver disease. The drug is not available in the United States.

Bromhexine has been studied in Europe with conflicting results. One study suggests that the drug is able to increase tear production and stability in SS, but has no apparent effect on oral symptoms. Another study found no difference in measurements of tear or saliva production between bromhexine and a placebo (inactive substance).

Few studies have been done on Efamol, a drug derived from evening primrose oil. This drug has been shown to increase some aspects of tear function, but not others, and it has not yet been shown to have any effect on saliva.

Additional studies have been proposed for all of these drugs.

Any form of salivary stimulation clearly requires the presence of at least a small amount of normal salivary gland tissue. Some patients with severe SS do not respond to any form of salivary stimulation.

Saliva substitutes. Several saliva substitutes that contain some

of the constituents of normal saliva are available commercially
(without prescription). Most of these are water-based and have a
short duration in the mouth, because they flow down the throat.
In controlled studies, these have been found to be more effective
than distilled water for relieving general symptoms of xerostomia
and more effective than a glycerine mouth rinse for relieving oral
discomfort at night.

Recently, gel-based preparations have been introduced that
may have longer duration in the mouth. Use of these preparations
may be helpful for patients with severe xerostomia, especially at
night, and for those wearing complete dentures. However, patients
with mild or even moderately severe xerostomia may find frequent
sips of water as effective. Oral lubricants containing lemon flavor
and citric acid to stimulate salivary flow have been suggested, but
these may have limited usefulness for patients with remaining natural teeth, because the acid can damage dental enamel.

SUMMARY

The treatment of xerostomia in patients with SS includes: (1)
preventing new and recurrent dental decay by frequent and regular
application of topical fluoride, remineralizing solutions, careful
dental supervision, and discontinuing sugar between meals; (2)
reducing oral symptoms by diagnosing and treating oral candidiasis, repeatedly if necessary; (3) stimulating the flow from salivary glands by taste simulation or other means; and (4) using some
form of saliva substitute, especially at night, and for patients wearing complete dentures, at any time.

6

Ears, Nose and Throat

Roger Miles Rose, M.D.

Gritty eyes. A dry, sore, sticky mouth and throat. A husky voice. A stopped-up, scabby, bloody nose. A diminished sense of smell and taste. Stuffy ears. Painful joints.

To Sjögren's syndrome (SS) patients, these symptoms may seem as awful as the plagues called down on Pharoah by Moses and may rob those who suffer from them of many of the comforts of life and the enjoyment of living.

Sjögren's syndrome affects more than the salivary and lacrimal (tear) glands and the joints. The mouth, pharynx (throat), larynx (voice box), nose, and ears are affected by dryness, too. Several parts of the body may suffer, as the autoimmune process progresses, gradually destroying the parotid, submandibular, and sublingual (major salivary) glands; drying up the hundreds of minor salivary glands in the lips, mouth, and throat; and also depriving the larynx and ears of needed moisture.

HOW IS THE MOUTH AFFECTED?

As the salivary glands lose their ability to produce saliva, the individual will experience xerostomia (dry mouth), often accompanied by burning and soreness. Constant thirst is a common complaint. Fissures (cracks) may develop at the corners of the lips, as they become irritated and raw from the lack of moisture. The tongue may become red or lumpy. Dental caries may be rampant, or difficulty in retaining dentures becomes evident. (The effects of Sjögren's syndrome on the teeth and other oral components of SS are discussed in Chapter 5.)

People with xerostomia are more likely to have oral candidiasis (a yeastlike fungal infection, such as thrush). This causes even more soreness and burning, red oral membranes, and occasionally white patches.

Affected individuals may notice a loss in the sense of taste, partly because the membranes in the mouth are dry and partly because dryness disrupts taste bud architecture and function.

HOW IS THE NOSE AFFECTED?

The thousands of tiny mucous glands in all areas of the nose are also damaged in Sjögren's syndrome. Nasal function includes cleansing and humidification of the air breathed. With dryness, the nose becomes congested and stuffy. As the dry crusts detach from the nasal membranes, occasional bleeding may be experienced. Although annoying, the bleeding is rarely severe. The drier and crustier the nose becomes, the less acute is the sense of smell.

HOW ARE THE EARS AFFECTED?

Just as Sjögren's syndrome damages the moisture-producing glands of the mouth and nose, it may also injure the mucous glands of the Eustachian tube (the tube running from the back of the nose to the middle ear). When this occurs, the ears may feel stuffy, and hearing acuity decreases. Should mucous glands within the middle ear itself become involved, middle ear infections may result. Fortunately, this does not happen very often in SS patients.

HOW IS THE LARYNX AFFECTED?

Mucous glands within the larynx are necessary for speaking. If the autoimmune disease atrophies these glands, the surface of the vocal cords will become dry, and thick clusters of mucus may stick to them. The voice will become husky, and one may find oneself constantly clearing the throat to dislodge the mucus. (Voice problems are thoroughly discussed in Chapter 19.)

HOW ARE THE SALIVARY GLANDS AFFECTED?

Often the first and most common symptom of Sjögren's syndrome is discomfort due to swelling of the major salivary glands (see illustration on page xxvii). The swelling is caused by infiltration of lymphocytes in these glands. Although these glands rarely become infected in SS, when they do, swelling is rapid and painful, accompanied by tenderness, fever, and possibly redness.

TESTS FOR SJOGREN'S SYNDROME

Some would argue that, because the diagnosis of Sjögren's syndrome can be made so readily on the basis of symptoms, diagnostic tests are unnecessary. Others ask: "Why bother testing patients who have dry eyes, dry mouth, swollen salivary glands, and rheumatoid arthritis? What else could it be but Sjögren's syndrome? And you're not going to treat these patients anyway."

But other diseases, such as sarcoidosis and tuberculosis, may cause the same galaxy of symptoms. These treatable disorders must be ruled out or managed. Moreover, as Sjögren's syndrome advances and becomes more troublesome, antimetabolite (cyclophosphamide or methotrexate, for example) and/or steroid therapy may help. But these therapies cannot be offered without a biopsy or blood tests to support the diagnosis of SS.

The following four tests *might* be performed or ordered by the otolaryngologist in evaluating a possible Sjögren's syndrome: (1)

lip biopsy; (2) sialography; (3) salivary gland scan; (4) salivary flow rate. (These tests are discussed in detail in Chapter 5.)

PRESCRIPTION TREATMENTS THAT STIMULATE SALIVA AND MUCUS

Unlike over-the-counter remedies that alleviate the symptoms of dryness, prescribed treatments are designed to stimulate saliva and mucus. Despite destruction of the secretory elements in the moisture-producing glands, enough function may remain to benefit from some form of stimulation.

Other medical conditions may make use of any of these prescription drugs inappropriate.

Systemic iodides, prescribed as either potassium iodide or as Organidin, help promote nasal and throat secretions. They are usually quite safe. Their side effects, however, include iodine allergy and stomach upset.

Pilocarpine is a potent stimulant of both the mucous glands and the salivary glands. It may be used either topically in the nose or taken by mouth. Because the range between efficacy and toxicity is narrow, this drug must be used under close medical supervision. Currently, studies are being conducted at the National Institute of Dental Research on the use of pilocarpine in treating xerostomia. (See *The Moisture Seekers Newsletter,* Vol. 3, No. 7 and No. 9.)

Nasalcrom, Vancenase, and *Nasalide* are well-tolerated prescription nasal sprays, when nasal allergy is thought to be part of the problem.

Guaifenesin, an expectorant, increases respiratory tract fluid secretions and helps to loosen phlegm and bronchial secretions. Guaifenesin, the main ingredient in Robitussin, is even more concentrated in Humibid LA, which is available by prescription.

MEDICATIONS AVAILABLE IN OTHER COUNTRIES

These medications have not been approved in the U. S., because their efficacy has not been demonstrated.

Bromhexine, a synthetic alkaloid, has been reported in two separate studies to increase tear and saliva flow. A third study showed no improvement. Although not available in the U. S., Bromhexine is sold as an over-the-counter drug in some European countries and Mexico.

Sialor (anetholetrithione), available in Canada, has been shown in some studies to be effective in treating dry mouth. Other investigators found it ineffective. It may cause gastric side effects.

OVER-THE-COUNTER (OTC) MEDICATIONS

For the ear: Dryness of ear canal skin, fairly common in Sjögren's syndrome, can be effectively treated by most emollients (skin softeners) or lubricants. Apply baby oil very gently with either a Q-tip or fingertips, inserted no more than one-half inch.

For the nose: Nasal dryness, stuffiness, and crusting can be alleviated by close attention with either OTC or home remedies. A mainstay of nasal hygiene is frequent use of a nasal douche. Saline solutions (Ocean, Nasal, Ayr, Salinex, to name a few) are readily available and come in a convenient squeeze bottle.

In place of saline, one might use Ringer's Lactate Solution, which can be obtained through surgical supply stores. Be sure to order it with a screw top.

Alkalol (not alcohol), diluted as directed on the bottle, is also very soothing and effective for relieving a dry, stuffy nose.

Since costs of these preparations mount quickly, one may wish to try making a nasal douche at home. (See Chapter 20 for complete instructions on nasal irrigation.)

Nasal Irrigator is a mechanical device for relieving dried up secretions in the nasal passages. This can be used as an attachment to either Puls-ator (Sears, Roebuck) or Water Pik. Nasal Irrigator can be ordered directly from Ethicare Products, P. O. Box 5027, Fort Lauderdale, FL 33310. (1988 cost: $17.95, including shipping and handling.)

Another device for irrigating the nasal passages is a plastic douche, which can be ordered from the Alkalol Co., Taunton, MA 02780.

In addition to nasal douching, nasal emollients are very desirable. Borofax, olive oil, vegetable oil, vitamin E oil, sweet almond oil, or petroleum jelly may be used on the lips and areas immediately adjacent inside the mouth. *To prevent pulmonary complications, these products should be applied very lightly and not poured into the nasal passages.*

When crusting becomes a significant problem, suggesting infection, OTC antibiotic ointments may be used. Either generic or brand names may be used, for example, Polymyxin, Bacitracin, Neomycin, and Neosporin.

When crusting is exceptionally troublesome, more active nasal douching may be used. Larger amounts of the homemade solution can be used and then expectorated. OTC Alkalol or Glycothymoline are effective and pleasantly aromatic douches. Use in half-strength concentrations. If they irritate, use weaker dilutions or return to the homemade saline solution.

For the mouth and throat: The addition of a teaspoon of glycerine to a glass of salt water makes a pleasant mouth wash and seems to stimulate secretions. Adding a teaspoonful of liquid Colace to this solution may make it even more effective as a gargle, because Colace's action on the surfaces of the mouth and throat may loosen some of the sticky secretions. Although Colace is well known for its anticonstipation benefits as well, there should be no concern about swallowing any of this solution when gargling. It may even benefit the lower throat.

(The dry mouth is thoroughly discussed in Chapter 5.)

ARE HUMIDIFIERS HELPFUL?

During warm weather months, which are associated in most areas of the country with a relatively high humidity, humidifiers are usually unnecessary. If the house or apartment seems too dry, its humidity can be measured.

Old-style humidifiers that use a belt and a drum that rotates in a bucket of water tend to collect infectious agents. They must be scrupulously cleaned every week with a weak bleach solution, following the manufacturer's instructions.

Newer-style ultrasonic humidifiers are quite effective. They also must be cleaned, not so much for fungi and mold spores as for mineral deposits.

(See also Chapter 15: "Allergy.")

AIR TRAVEL

Unfortunately, aircraft interiors are significantly drier than even most steam-heated homes. Together with the exceedingly poor ventilation systems on most airplanes, this very dry air can cause significant distress to the Sjögren's syndrome patient. When flying, keep the nasal membranes constantly moistened by spraying with saline solution. A glass of nonalcoholic fluid should be consumed every half hour.

7

Gastrointestinal Tract

Seymour Katz, M.D.
Kenneth Nyer, M.D.

Since xerostomia (dry mouth) was first described as a characteristic feature of Sjögren's syndrome (SS), other gastrointestinal manifestations have been noted in the literature. They include: esophageal webs and motility disorders, which result in difficulty in swallowing; achlorhydria (gastric acid deficiency); chronic gastritis (stomach inflammation); pancreatic disease; and liver disease.

Many of these disorders were felt to occur simultaneously with SS and were conjectured to be due to similar immunologic mechanisms or as a consequence of the sicca complex (dryness).

On their first visit to a new doctor, people with Sjögren's syndrome would do well to identify themselves as SS patients. They should be prepared for an honest response from the doctor, who might say, "I don't know anything about Sjögren's syndrome." Rather than becoming discouraged, the patient should remember that he or she is an important source of information for the medical professional. If the patient works along with an interested doctor, both will benefit.

XEROSTOMIA

Although this topic is dealt with in detail in Chapter 5, saliva production is an integral part of digestion and requires a brief discussion here. Without saliva, food cannot be softened or broken into particles small enough to swallow. Saliva is needed not only for chewing properly, but for moving food effectively to the back of the mouth, where it triggers the swallowing reflex. Saliva is absolutely essential for lubricating food as it passes down the esophagus (food tube) to the stomach.

In addition to serving as a lubricant, saliva also serves a local protective function, not only for the mucous membranes of the mouth, but also for the teeth and other structures in the mouth and throat.

There are six major salivary glands and many minor ones. The parotid glands account for 25% of secretion. The other major salivary glands account for an additional 70%. A normal adult produces 1.5 liters of saliva daily. Most of this occurs during eating.

Sjögren's syndrome patients often complain of dysphagia (difficulty in swallowing). They also find eating difficult, because of an uncomfortable parched red mouth. Burning of the mouth or prickling sensations may occur. There also may be a metallic taste associated with SS, as well as with other disorders, which is as yet unexplained.

Adequate lubrication of the mouth with water or other fluids and avoiding dehydration will help control much of the dysphagia. Drugs that can lead to dry mouth, such as antispasmodics (atropine derivatives), decongestants (Sudafed), and antihistamines (Dimetapp) should be avoided.

ARTIFICIALLY SWEETENED CANDIES
MAY CAUSE ABDOMINAL DISTRESS

In their attempt to keep their mouths moist by ingesting dietetic gums and candies, Sjögrens's syndrome patients may experience abdominal bloating, diarrhea, and cramps, following excessive use of these artifically sweetened gums and candies.

Should these symptoms occur, the patient must consult his or her physician and have a full physical examination and laboratory evaluation. Before embarking on a long and costly path of endless exams, some dietary adjustments and careful discussions with one's physician may shed light on this increasingly recognized disorder.

POSTCRICOID WEBS

Postcricoid webs are bandlike narrowings of the esophagus behind the cartilage of the larynx (voice box). For about 50% of patients, these bands usually lead to difficulty in swallowing solid foods.

Symptomless webs have been identified in 10% of normal individuals. Postcricoid webs have been found in patients with SS, but are also associated with iron deficiency anemia, ulcerative colitis, and thyroid disease.

This narrowing of the esophagus is diagnosed by cinefluorography (x-rays taken during swallowing) or by direct visualization of the esophagus with a fiberoptic endoscope. In an x-ray, webs appear as rings of wavelike material in the esophagus.

If symptomatic, webs can be stretched or treated by rupture with a rubber device passed into the esophagus.

ESOPHAGEAL DYSMOTILITY

Esophageal dysmotility means abnormal motion of the esophagus and is characterized by an abnormality in the normal wavelike contractions of the esophagus called peristalsis.

Reduced muscle tone in the wall of the esophagus leads to reflux of gastric juice, producing a burning sensation behind the breastbone (heartburn), difficulty in swallowing, and chest pain. Prolonged reflux of acid results in a chronic irritation known as esophagitis.

Because burning, chest pain, and chest pressure may be symptomatic of heart disease, these symptoms should be checked out by an internist or cardiologist, before the patient sees a gastroenterologist.

Some investigators believe that esophageal dysmotility may be an inherent muscle disorder, unrelated to dryness or a moisture deficiency. This is controversial. Recent studies indicate that lack of moisture plays an important part. Other work indicates there may be true inflammation of the muscles of the esophagus. This is not yet fully understood. There may be some inflammation of the glands of the esophagus, but this is still conjecture.

The diagnosis is made by esophageal motility studies, that is, by manometry (pressure studies) and by simultaneous monitoring of the acid content of the esophagus. In some instances, x-ray studies show abnormal contractions of the esophagus, while motility studies may reveal markedly increased pressure. Sometimes, it is necessary to detect these abnormalities by provocation with cold water or chemical stimulation.

A diagnosis of Sjögren's syndrome does not necessarily mean that swallowing symptoms are due to esophageal dysmotility. Obstruction, gastric-peptic problems, strictures, webs, and growths must be ruled out.

Treatment is directed toward relaxing the smooth muscle of the esophagus. Nitroglycerin and calcium channel blockers may be helpful. If medication does not give relief, the esophagus may be dilated (widened) by passage of a soft tube through the mouth. Longitudinal myotomy (surgery of the tightened muscles) has also been used, but only in the most difficult cases.

Patients with heartburn usually have an increased production of saliva due to acid stimulation. Normally, the increased saliva serves to dilute the acid. However, this is not true in Sjögren's syndrome patients, who are more prone to heartburn, because of their inability to produce enough saliva to offset the irritating effects of acid. Taking water alone, instead of antacid preparations, might relieve heartburn. Water dilutes the acid and makes the esophagus empty better.

ACHALASIA

Several children with juvenile Sjögren's syndrome have been reported to have achalasia, a muscle disorder of the lower esophagus. Achalasia is unusual in adults with SS. The disorder consists of a motor abnormality with incomplete relaxation of the lower esophageal sphincter muscle. In addition, normal peristaltic contraction to swallowing is absent. The result of these abnormalities leads to megaesophagus (marked widening of the esophagus).

The symptoms of achalasia are similar to those of esophageal dysmotility, namely, progressive difficulty in swallowing, weight loss of long duration, and pain following eating. Many patients present themselves to an internist or pulmonary specialist, because fluid does not go down the esophagus, but spills over into the lungs, particularly at night. This causes nocturnal chest pains and cough, with unexpected bronchitis or persistent pneumonia.

The diagnosis of achalasia is dependent on x-ray studies.

Drug treatment is usually not effective. Dilation of the narrowed sphincter is required.

SS patients with achalasia may have an associated decrease in stomach acid secretion. No one knows why, but some physicians think decreased acid production is caused by a mechanical irritation of the dry esophageal mucous membrances by swallowed food.

ACHLORHYDRIA/CHRONIC ATROPHIC GASTRITIS

One of the more common gastrointestinal diseases found in Sjögren's syndrome patients is chronic atrophic gastritis, or irritation of the stomach unrelated to excess acid. SS patients have decreased acid, a condition known as achlorhydria. All the Maalox, Mylanta, and Tagamet will do absolutely nothing to help.

Decreased acid and lymphocytic infiltration of the stomach are found in many SS patients. This has been confirmed by detecting low acid secretion in the stomach. Antibodies to cells that secrete acid have been found in the serum of SS patients. The cause is thought to be autoimmune in nature.

Chronic atrophic gastritis is longstanding inflammation of the stomach. Published reports show a low blood level of pepsinogen, an enzyme of digestion activated by gastric acid, and a high level of gastrin, a substance that ordinarily stimulates gastric acid secretion. In SS patients, the gastrin is unable to stimulate gastric acid secretion.

Symptoms include nausea and upper abdominal pain.

Endoscopy (visualization of the stomach with a fiberoptic endoscope), accompanied by an endoscopic biopsy of the stomach, are often used to make the diagnosis.

Infiltration of the gastric lining with lymphocytes (white blood cells), similar to the involvement of the salivary glands in SS, has been thought to be a contributing cause of chronic atrophic gastritis.

This does not mean that Sjögren's syndrome causes chronic atrophic gastritis. Age probably plays a contributing role, since approximately 41% of patients between 41 and 65 years of age have variable levels of atrophic gastritis. However, this does not account for the 81% incidence of atrophic gastritis reported in SS. Other coexistent autoimmune diseases and medications may play a role.

Despite a great deal of elegant research, there has been no success in various forms of treatment of atrophic gastritis with decreased production of acid. Poor vitamin B12 absorption will occur in patients without gastric acid. This may result in a form of anemia. Anemia due to iron deficiency may also be associated with chronic gastritis. Iron and vitamin B12 replacement are usually required for these individuals.

PANCREATIC DISEASE

Since Sjögren's syndrome is a disease of secretory glands, glandular organs associated with the gastrointestinal tract are often involved. Pancreatic insufficiency indicates the failure of the pancreas to secrete its digestive enzymes. Diarrhea and steatorrhea (greasy stools) are common symptoms.

In SS patients, diarrhea may arise from a number of sources and should not be treated routinely with paregoric or Lomotil. The cause must be determined before it can be treated intelligently.

The treatment for pancreatic enzyme insufficiency requires the administration of oral pancreatic enzymes, often in high dosage, and decreasing gastric acid with a drug, such as cimetidine (Tagamet), unless gastric acid deficiency is already present.

Acute pancreatitis, or inflammation of the pancreas, has been rarely described in SS patients. Pancreatitis presents with abdominal pain and abdominal tenderness. This usually occurs in the upper abdomen with radiation to the back. Persistent, unrelenting nausea and vomiting are also prominent. Laboratory tests show an elevated serum enzyme, amylase, which is characteristic of this disease.

The treatment of acute pancreatitis is similar to that of pancreatitis of other causes. This includes analgesics for pain and intravenous fluids.

Amylase is produced by the salivary glands, as well as by the pancreas. Although they are distinctly different, a hospital emergency room may measure the amylase level of an accident victim without defining its origin. In an SS patient, the test results could be misinterpreted as pancreatitis. Therefore, SS patients should have a standard amylase test performed when they are well. If the level is elevated, it should be further studied, so that the patient and his or her physicians know whether the elevation is from the salivary glands or the pancreas.

LIVER DISEASE

Autoimmune liver diseases are commonly found in association with Sjögren's syndrome. These consist of primary biliary cirrhosis, chronic active hepatitis, and cryptogenic cirrhosis. In studies of SS patients, approximately one-fifth were found to have enlarged livers and cirrhosis was occasionally demonstrated.

The diseases discussed here are considered to be mediated by autoimmune mechanisms.

PRIMARY BILIARY CIRRHOSIS

Primary biliary cirrhosis is an impairment of bile excretion caused by autoimmune inflammation around bile ducts of the liver, small channels that transport bile into the intestine. Patients have symptoms related to backup of bile acids and salts, namely, itching, dark urine, pale stools, jaundice, excess fat in the stool, and cholesterol deposits under the skin, known as xanthomas. Most cases occur in middle-aged women.

The association with the sicca complex suggests a common immunological mechanism. The finding of antimitochondrial antibodies, antibodies against mitochondria (a cell component) in the blood, is diagnostic of primary biliary cirrhosis. The diagnosis is made by analysis of all symptoms, positive antimitochondrial antibodies, and liver biopsy.

Other causes of bile duct obstruction must be excluded, especially those easily treated, such as a gallstone. X-ray studies, done either by placing a thin needle into the liver or by endoscopy, may be required to evaluate the bile ducts.

The treatment of primary biliary cirrhosis is limited to controlling symptoms. No therapy has been found to stem the natural progression of the disease. The resultant itching, which can occur anywhere in the body, can be treated with lotions, phenobarbital, steroids, or cholestyramine, a resin that binds cholesterol and bile salts. Fat-soluble vitamins—A, D, and K—should be given to prevent weakening of bones and bleeding disorders.

CHRONIC ACTIVE HEPATITIS

Chronic active hepatitis is a process of continuing autoimmune inflammation and scarring, which may lead to cirrhosis of the liver. This disease is usually a result of infection with a hepatitis virus, a reaction to specific drugs, or secondary to certain inherited liver diseases.

Evidence of an autoimmune disorder is the finding of antibodies in the blood directed against mitochondria, smooth muscle, and thyroid.

Typical symptoms of fatigue, jaundice, malaise, anorexia, and low-grade fever are common.

The diagnosis is usually confirmed by liver biopsy.

Steroids (cortisone) have been used to treat this disorder in selected symptomatic patients.

CRYPTOGENIC CIRRHOSIS

Cryptogenic cirrhosis is a chronic liver disorder associated with enhanced formation of connective tissue in the liver. As with chronic active hepatitis, viral hepatitis is thought to be an initiating factor.

The same symptoms that occur with active hepatitis may be seen. Abdominal pain and ascites (a fluid collection in the abdomen) may be present and may progress to encephalopathy (an altered mental status) in this as in other liver diseases.

Treatment is limited to supportive care, controlling ascites, diet, and prompt treatment of infections.

Again, the underlying cause is thought to be an autoimmune mechanism. Conceivably, both these liver disorders and multisymtemic diseases, such as SS, are the result of viral infection or toxic agents.

CELIAC DISEASE (GLUTEN ENTEROPATHY)

Several patients with Sjögren's syndrome have been described with celiac disease (gluten intolerance). Celiac disease is caused by gluten, a grain constituent, which in certain people causes damage to the small intestine. It is thought that an immune hypersensitivity to gluten results in celiac disease.

The intestinal damage results in malabsorption (poor absorption of food nutrients from the bowel), leading to diarrhea and vitamin deficiencies.

The diagnosis of celiac disease requires an intestinal biopsy, as well as blood, urine, and stool studies documenting malabsorption.

Treatment consists of a gluten-free diet and replacement of vitamins and minerals.

SUMMARY

Sjögren's syndrome is a complex disease, involving the entire body and often the gastrointestinal tract. The common features of the gastrointestinal manifestations of SS are lymphocytic infiltrates of organs and circulating antibodies in the blood. Lymphocytes found in people with dry mouth and gastric problems indicate that these people may have SS, also. Autoantibodies have routinely been found in patients with achlorhydria, hepatitic disease, and celiac disease. The common factor in all these disorders appears to be their autoimmune nature.

8

Vagina

John J. Willems, M.D.

When a rheumatologist refers a woman with Sjögren's syndrome (SS) to a gynecologist for evaluation, her problem is usually vaginal dryness and dyspareunia (painful intercourse), caused by a lack of lubrication. Vulvar discomfort and vaginal yeast infections are also common in women with SS.

Many women with Sjögren's syndrome do have adequate vaginal lubrication. On the other hand, vaginal dryness, vulvar discomfort, and yeast infections are common problems in women who do not have SS. So the situation is not necessarily related to dry eyes and dry mouth. The first step in the gynecological examination is to rule out other causes of these symptoms.

Although many women with Sjögren's syndrome are no longer interested in bearing children, questions do arise concerning SS and obstetrical risks. From women at the other end of the reproductive age range, gynecologists receive questions about the use of estrogen in postmenopausal women with autoimmune disease.

WOMEN WITH SS HAVE SPECIAL PROBLEMS

Sjögren's syndrome is not the uncommon problem that many have been taught to believe. This disorder, including primary Sjögren's syndrome and SS in association with other autoimmune diseases, may be the second most common rheumatologic disease in the United States. Up to 30% of people with rheumatoid arthritis, 10% of those with systemic lupus erythematosus (SLE), and 1% of scleroderma patients have secondary SS. No one understands why SS predominantly affects women, usually in their third or fourth decades of life.

Women with Sjögren's syndrome not only have special obstetrical and gynecological (OB/GYN) problems, but very little has been written about them. In a recent on-line search of the medical literature over the past five years, no articles were found on the treatment of painful intercourse in women with SS.

RULING OUT OTHER CAUSES

Before the gynecologist can attribute vaginal dryness to Sjögren's syndrome, other causes must first be ruled out.

At menopause, for example, decreased estrogen levels may lead to vaginal symptoms, as does surgical removal of the ovaries, the predominant source of estrogen.

Vaginal infections often cause discomfort during and after intercourse. Chronic diseases, such as diabetes and systemic lupus erythematosus, may cause a lack of lubrication. This may be compounded by the debilitating nature of the disease, which can lead to a loss of sexual interest.

Previous painful intercourse can inhibit lubrication, when the woman anticipates another painful experience. Lack of adequate sexual stimulation for whatever reasons can also lead to limited lubrication.Various pelvic pathologies, for example, ovarian tumors and uterine fibroids, can cause vaginal dryness and painful intercourse secondarily.

HOW ARE GYNECOLOGIC
PROBLEMS IN SS TREATED?

Once other causes of vaginal dryness and painful intercourse have been investigated and ruled out, a true relationship to Sjögren's syndrome may be inferred. The woman and her partner need to be reassured that this is a physiological problem and is not related to a failure of sexual arousal.

To replace normal vaginal lubrication, sterile, greaseless lubricants are helpful. The internal use of preparations containing petrolatum or oils that seal in moisture, such as Vaseline or cocoa butter, should be avoided.

Only water-soluble lubricants should be used in the vagina, because oil-based lubricants foil the vagina's natural self-cleansing mechanism. Oil-based lubricants are also fairly immune to douches. Moreover, oil-based lubricants can trap natural moisture in the vagina and cause maceration of the sensitive vaginal tissues. They have been implicated in some allergic problems. Because they impair sperm mobility, they are specifically contraindicated for the couple trying to conceive.

One must be careful, when it comes to advertising and vaginal preparations. Madison Avenue has been touting certain lubricants as "personal lubricants," with overtones of enhanced sexual fulfillment. However, any lubricant with a color, taste, or any other additive is not the right one for most women, and certainly not the right one, if their vaginal dryness is related to Sjögren's syndrome.

The ideal lubricant is colorless, odorless, tasteless, water-soluble, and of a consistency that allows it to remain in the vagina.

If too much lubricant is used, the result is frictionless and rather messy coitus. If this is a persistent problem, a woman might consider using a minimum of vaginal gel or cream and then adding a thin layer directly to the penis.

For those women dissatisfied with K-Y Jelly or H-R Lubricating Jelly, a trial of Surgilube (E. Fougera & Co., Melville, NY 11747) or Maxilube (Mission Pharmacal Co., San Antonio, TX 78296) may be attempted. Some women find Maxilube's somewhat thicker consistency markedly preferable.

Cortisone creams are not good for vaginal dryness.

When the lack of lubrication is caused by decreased estrogen, either at menopause or following surgical removal of the ovaries, this can be corrected with appropriate estrogen replacement. For vaginal yeast infections, prompt treatment with clotrimazole cream or suppositories (Gyne-Lotrimin) is effective and safe.

Dry external vulvar surfaces may be treated with lubricating creams, as you would any other skins surfaces. Some women find a light lubricating oil, such as vitamin E oil, useful.

Treatment of Sjögren's-related gynecologic problems is symptomatic only. No cure has yet been found for the underlying disease. With personal testing and compassionate gynecologic care, the SS patient can find what works best for her.

OBSTETRICAL RISKS

The association between maternal antibodies to SS-A/Ro and SS-B/La and congenital heart block is disscussed in Chapter 16. A brief review of the obstetrical risks is presented here.

Obstetrical authorities report higher rates of recurrent abortion, fetal death, and congenital heart block in pregnancies complicated by maternal autoimmune disease. (Congenital heart block is a dysfunction of the rate/rhythm conduction system in the fetal or infant heart, leading to an abnormal heart rate or rhythm.)

Although SLE is the autoimmune disease most often associated with obstetrical problems, the relationship of Sjögren's syndrome and SLE may be closer than previously appreciated, particularly when one considers the similarities in autoantibodies detected by laboratory techniques.

Certain autoantibodies, such as antinuclear antibodies (ANAs) and antibodies against SS-A or Ro, have been implicated in congenital heart block. These antibodies are found in 50% to 70% of SS patients. Approximately 5% of women with these antibodies have an infant with congenital heart block. The precise likelihood of a child having congenital heart block, when the mother has these antibodies, has not been determined. It is probably no more than one in 20 and no less than one in 60, with no history of a previously affected infant.

The most striking antibody association is between pregnancy

loss and antiphospholipid antibodies, lupus anticoagulant, and anticardiolipin. These autoantibodies have been identified in patients with SLE and other autoimmune disorders, as well as in patients with no apparent disease.

Because of these associations, all women with SS or SLE, in addition to women who have had recurrent spontaneous abortions or a false positive blood test for syphilis, should have autoantibody screening and appropriate counselling before becoming pregnant. These pregnancies require high risk obstetrical care and consultation with an obstetrical specialist or perinatologist.

A team approach, combining both rheumatology and obstetrics, will optimize the outcome for both mother and baby. The role of the rheumatologist in helping to prevent complications is discussed in Chapter 16.

SJOGREN'S SYNDROME AND MENOPAUSE

Women with Sjögrens's syndrome often wonder if an autoimmune disease precludes the use of postmenopausal estrogen replacement therapy (ERT).

As pointed out, estrogen taken orally or applied locally is very useful in treating postmenopausal vaginal dryness and painful intercourse. Unless there is an underlying medical contraindication, such as a history of breast cancer, estrogen/progestin replacement therapy is often recommended for postmenopausal patients.

Currently, analysis of the benefits versus the risks of ERT indicates a major benefit in preventing osteoporosis. There is also recent suggestive evidence that ERT may lower a woman's overall risk of cardiovascular disease. There does not appear to be an associated elevation of blood pressure on the lower dosages now used.

9

Skin

Charles S. Baraf, M.D.

People with Sjögren's syndrome (SS) commonly notice many kinds of skin changes. They may experience dry skin, small white bumps that peel, red spots, chapped lips, cracked fingertips, brittle nails, flushing, and hair loss, as well as darkening or lightening of the skin.

The largest organ in the body, the skin is normally moisturized by the many glands within it that secrete oil and water. When the water-producing sweat glands are working, the moisture they provide is evaporated, cooling the body. Although their primary purpose is regulation of body temperature, the sweat glands also supply moisture for the skin itself, keeping it healthy.

Sjögren's syndrome frequently affects these glands, as well as those that produce saliva and tears. When the sweat glands are not functioning, the skin becomes like the earth during a drought, turning dry, brittle, cracked, and losing its ability to retain moisture. Between one-third and two-thirds of people with SS have problems with dry skin.

A type of "hot flash" or flushing experienced by Sjögren's syndrome patients is also caused by malfunctioning sweat glands. Without temperature-regulating moisture, the body can easily become flushed or chilled. Emotional factors aggravate this problem, but are not the cause.

HOW TO ADD MOISTURE TO THE SKIN

Paradoxically, because it evaporates on the skin, water causes dryness. Therefore, people with Sjögren's syndrome should avoid frequent or long hot baths and showers. Since the skin does a good job of cleaning itself, daily baths are not always necessary. Those who feel more comfortable bathing every day should take a "quickie" shower and then "damp dry," that is, blot the water from the body very lightly with a towel, leaving a thin film of moisture on the skin.

While the skin is still damp, apply a moisturizer. Despite contrary reports, no drug or cream is yet known that will stimulate the glands in the skin to produce more oil or water. All moisturizers are equally effective—even Crisco, if one can tolerate the smell—so there is no need to buy fancy or expensive creams.

Petroleum jelly (Vaseline) and products containing urea (Carmol) do a good job. Dermatologists and other physicians treat difficult or stubborn cases of dryness with a prescription preparation containing 12% lactate.

Creams work much better than lotions. The reason for this is that lotions are made of of chemicals interspersed in a liquid. The liquid evaporates, leaving patches of concentrated chemicals on the skin. A cream, on the other hand, is greasier and more readily absorbed. The greasier the cream, the better for the skin. Use whatever cream works best, avoiding anything that causes a sensitivity reaction.

Not only does water dry the skin, but soaps, being defatting agents, dry it further. A good substitute is Cetaphil lotion, which is available over the counter. Rather than removing makeup with soap, use anything that does not cause more dryness or sensitivity. Experiment and find out what works best.

Many SS patients suffer from painful cracks at the corners of the mouth and inflamed lips. Cracked lips may result when saliva causes an overgrowth of yeast. As part of aging, the angles of the skin lines around the mouth change, accentuating these cracks. A good way to alleviate dry lips is applying a thin coating of Vaseline or Crisco on them at night. Yeast overgrowth is treated with anti-fungal medications.

WATCH OUT FOR THE WEATHER

Just as the rest of the body is dressed for various kinds of weather, so the exposed areas of the skin must be weatherproofed.

Eczema, sometimes caused by allergy, can develop from weather conditions and dryness.

Weather exacerbates painful cracks around the fingernails, even in people who do not have SS. Unfortunately, nothing works very well to prevent this. Frequent use of a hand cream containing urea will soften the skin and alleviate the pain.

In winter, notorious for drying out the skin, liberal applications of moisturizer are needed.

RAYNAUD'S PHENOMENON

Raynaud's phenomenon, a condition commonly seen in connective tissue diseases, including SS, affects the small blood vessels of the hands and feet. The blood vessels go into spasm, resulting in pain, numbness, and blanching of the extemities when exposed to cold. If this phenomenon is present, it is important to protect the hands and feet against cold temperatures. Gloves must be worn when handling foods from the freezer. Some patients are treated with calcium antagonist drugs, such as nifedipine (Procardia).

THE SUN CAN BE AN ENEMY

In summer, spend no more than 20 minutes a day in the sun. If one must remain outdoors longer, protection with a sunscreen and a hat is essential.

Sun exposure is not good for anyone, not only because the sun is a drying agent, but because it produces delayed effects. Fairer people are more sensitive to sun damage than those who are darker skinned. The dramatic increase in skin cancer, especially life-threatening melanoma, is directly related to exposure to sunlight.

Like many forms of cancer, melanoma is a preventable disease. The earlier it is diagnosed, the easier it is to cure. The more superficial the tumor, the better the prognosis. For early discovery, look for the four (ABCD) signs of melanoma:

(1) Asymmetry: A melanoma tends to have an asymmetrical shape, while a mole is usually symmetrical.

(2) Border: Melanomas typically have an irregular, notched border.

(3) Color: A melanoma is variegated, going from black to brown, to white, to blue, to gray. Any multicolored mole is suspicious.

(4) Diameter: A normal mole is usually 5 mm. (about 1/4 inch) across.

Any mole that changes should be brought to the attention of a physician.

Some people with Sjögren's syndrome have either an increase or a loss of pigmentation. No one knows why.

Sunlight promotes hyperpigmentation or the production of melanin, the compound responsible for coloring the skin. Hyperpigmentation is commonly called a suntan. In hypopigmentation, the skin loses its color in affected areas.

Injuries to the skin can either leave it unaffected, or cause the skin to get darker, or cause it to lose pigment through loss of pigment cells. Vitiligo, a loss of pigment with no known underlying disorder, may be similar to other autoimmune diseases, since patients frequently have detectable antibodies. Certain drugs, called psoralens, sensitize the skin to the effects of sunlight. In turn, this stimulates pigment cells. While this treatment is effective, many sessions are needed over a long period of time.

Whether the person with Sjögren's syndrome has a loss or an increase of pigmentation, exposure to the sun will make it worse. If a pigmentation problem is present, a sunscreen is a must. Those rated #15 provide good coverage. Higher coverages are more expensive, but not more effective.

Paraminobenzoic acid (PABA), the most common ingredient in sunscreens, causes an allergic reaction in some people. People who are allergic to sulfa should not use PABA sunscreens. Effective sunscreens without PABA are: Ti-Screen, Solbar PF, and Red Veterinary Petrolatum (RVP). Sometimes, a component in the sunscreen base is the culprit in sensitivity, rather than the active ingredient. Oral PABA is not effective as a sunscreen.

Since most sunscreens are water-soluble, reapplication after swimming is necessary.

HAIR LOSS

To their dismay, many people with Sjögren's syndrome and lupus lose their hair, especially after an acute flare-up. Hair loss may follow a high fever, surgery, general anesthesia, childbirth, or any other shock to the system.

The average human scalp contains about 100,000 hairs. Only 80% to 90% of these hairs are growing. The remainder, those that have completed their growth cycle and are in the process of dying, are in a resting phase. Normally, about 100 hairs a day are lost, but since new hair is growing all the time, the loss is not noticed. Since a resting hair takes about three months to fall out, hair loss caused by a shock to the system will not be noticed until about three months after a trauma or flare-up of SS.

People with SS or lupus lose their hair in patches. Called *alopecia,* this type of fallout is caused by a destruction of hair follicles. Although some cases of baldness respond to treatment with Minoxidil, a blood pressure drug found to stimulate hair growth, Minoxidil has no effect on hair loss due to inflammatory destruction of hair follicles. The patchy hair loss of SS is treated with various methods, including cortisone injections.

OTHER SKIN PROBLEMS

Some people with Sjögren's syndrome get a condition called *exfoliative dermatitis,* which causes fever, chills, and red skin that peels. Others get *acne rosacea,* resulting in a red nose and redness in other parts of the body. Caused by an inflammation of the skin's oil-producing glands, this condition can be aggravated by alcohol and hot drinks, which dilate the blood vessels. As one grows older, the foundation around blood vessels becomes weaker, frequently causing black and blue marks.

Purpura, caused by blood escaping from a blood vessel into the skin, look similar to a bruise. Unlike bruises, purpura can always be felt. They are a hallmark of vasculitis, inflammation of a blood vessel, another condition that is frequent in SS and connective tissue diseases. A more detailed discussion of vasculitis appears in Chapter 13.

Due to dryness of the skin and inflammation of the blood vessels, wounds heal slowly in SS patients. However, most authorities do not believe vitamin E helps heal wounds.

WHAT TO AVOID

While people with Sjögren's syndrome can help their skin by adding moisture, they can also prevent problems by avoiding certain things, among them cortisone creams, collagen injections, and the vitamin A derivatives called retinoids.

Cortisone creams cause weakening of the skin and blood vessels, accentuating the thinness of the skin. This is already a problem in people with SS. Therefore, even over-the-counter cortisone creams, which are quite mild, should be used with discretion.

Sjögren's syndrome patients should also avoid collagen injections. The collagen used in these cosmetic treatments comes from cows and is therefore a foreign agent. Since the bodies of people with SS are already reacting to their own cells, they don't need an invasion of foreign militia.

Vitamin A derivatives, called retinoids, are receiving a lot of attention lately. A form of retinoid called Retin-A, containing the acid form of vitamin A, is called retinoic acid (Tretinoin). Effective in treating bad cases of acne, Retin-A is now being used for other purposes, such as minimizing wrinkles. (It will not make wrinkles disappear.)

Until studies of the long-term effects of these substances have been completed, they should not be widely used. Because retinoids can be irritating, especially to fair-skinned people, SS patients should avoid them.

Like other people with chronic conditons, SS patients should beware of fancy marketing claims. For any skin problem except dryness, it is important that a dermatologist be consulted. SS patients should not attempt to treat these problems themselves.

Part III

Extraglandular Involvement

10

Connective Tissue Diseases

Harry Spiera, M.D.

Some people who suffer from the dry eyes or dry mouth of Sjö-gren's syndrome (SS) are also troubled by swollen, red, hot, and tender joints; joint pain without swelling; muscle pain and weakness; skin rashes; or symptoms of major organ dysfunction. These patients may be classified as having secondary Sjögren's syndrome. Patients who are diagnosed as secondary SS have dry eyes or dry mouth in association with an underlying disorder, usually one of the connective tissue diseases.

Connective tissue diseases are those involving the tissues that seem to hold the various organs together, among them the bones, muscles, tendons, ligaments, and a component called ground substance. The connective tissue diseases most commonly associated with Sjögren's syndrome are rheumatoid arthritis (RA), systemic lupus erythematosus (SLE), scleroderma, and dermatomyositis (DM).

COMMON FACTORS

While each of these disorders has features of autoimmunity, the causes of all of these diseases are unknown. Our knowledge of them is mainly descriptive. In each, doctors know something about the patterns of involvement, the type of symptoms produced, the kinds of tissues involved, and some of the characteristic abnormalities in blood tests. These help the physician make a diagnosis.

All of these diseases are chronic and unpredictable. They may improve spontaneously. Patients experience varying degrees of illness and disability. Sjögren's syndrome more or less complicates any of these illnesses. In some patients, SS itself becomes the cardinal problem.

The physician who cares for patients with various connective tissue diseases must be alert for the symptoms and manifestations of Sjögren's syndrome. While there are treatments for all of these diseases, cures have not yet been found.

Treatments directed at Sjögren's syndrome, whether associated with a connective tissue disease or not, are discussed in other chapters of this book. They are not the same as treatments for the various connective tissue diseases described here.

RHEUMATOID ARTHRITIS (RA)

Rheumatoid arthritis is mainly a disease of the joints. For unknown reasons, the joints become inflamed and painfully swollen, red, hot, and tender. Although any joint in the body may be involved, the metacarpophalangeal and proximal interphalangeal joints of the hands (knuckles), wrists, elbows, shoulders, knees, ankles, and feet are the joints usually affected by RA.

This extremely common disease afflicts about 1% of the population, women more frequently than men. Rheumatoid arthritis can occur at any age. An estimated 250,000 children in the United States alone have RA. At the other end of the spectrum, patients in their 90s may suffer from acute RA.

The course of rheumatoid arthritis is unpredictable. Some patients have short-lived, acute attacks and then get better. Others go on to a chronic, progressive disease, leading to joint damage and destruction. Many patients experience RA as an illness in which many episodes of marked inflammation alternate with episodes of feeling much better.

Because spontaneous remission is part of the natural course of the disease, some patients attribute their improvement to treatments that have no value. If, for example, spontaneous remission follows visiting a radioactive mine in Utah, eating a diet of peanut butter or mushrooms, wearing a copper bracelet, or doing any of numerous things that have been advocated for the treatment of RA, these patients may mistake their remission for a cure, crediting whatever "treatment" preceded it.

For this reason, medical specialists insist that any arthritis treatment be subjected to a double-blind study, one in which neither the physicians nor the patients being treated know whether the patients are receiving the active ingredient being tested or a placebo (an inactive substance).

If medical investigators can show on objective measurements (measurements that can be evaluated independently) that patients receiving the active ingredient do better than those taking the placebo, then that treatment can be said to be successful to some degree. Few medicines have met this rigid test.

Although rheumatoid arthritis primarily involves joints, it is a generalized illness that can affect several organ systems. Many RA patients have anemia and fever and are easily fatigued. On occasion, RA may affect the heart, lungs, nerves, skin, and eyes. In a significant number of patients, RA is associated with inflammation of salivary and lacrimal glands. These patients have secondary Sjögren's syndrome.

Rheumatoid arthritis is treated in several ways. For some patients, rest, a range-of-motion exercise program, and aspirin to relieve pain and swelling are all that is necessary. If the disease becomes more severe or progressive, the physician will prescribe nonsteroidal anti-inflammatory agents.

In some cases, doctors use medicines that seem to have the capacity to stop the illness, rather than just relieve symptoms. These medicines include gold, d-penicillamine, the antimalarial drugs (quinine derivatives first developed to treat malaria), and immunosuppressive agents. All of these medicines have potentially serious side effects. Their use must be monitored by a physician well acquainted with these drugs.

Cortisone, very effective in reducing inflammation, is often administered either by mouth or by injection directly into the joint to suppress pain, swelling, and inflammation. However, like all powerful medicines, cortisone has potential side effects. The physician must weigh the potential benefits against the potential risks for the individual patient.

Physical therapy is often part of the therapeutic program. This includes various modalities to relieve pain and exercise programs to preserve range of motion and strengthen muscles. Should the illness become progressive and cause significant joint destruction, orthopedic surgeons have made much progress in replacing damaged joints.

In some patients with Sjögren's syndrome secondary to rheumatoid arthritis, an improvement in the RA may be accompanied by an improvement in SS symptoms as well. This may be related to a stopping of the progression of dryness in various areas of the body. At other times, the rheumatoid arthritis is kept under control, but the SS symptoms tend to progress and worsen.

SYSTEMIC LUPUS ERYTHEMATOSUS (SLE)

Although systemic lupus erythematosus is predominantly an illness of young women of childbearing age, it can affect almost any age group and occurs in men as well.

SLE has many manifestations associated with a variety of autoantibodies. Proteins are formed that have the capacity of reacting with the body's own constituents.

Virtually any part of the body can be involved in SLE. The illness can vary from a very mild disease, in which the patient has nothing more than some fatigue and joint discomfort, but no serious organ involvement, to one that involves virtually every organ system and can lead to death. With earlier diagnosis and more effective treatments, SLE mortality has decreased markedly over the last 10 years.

Many patients have joint pains, with or without swelling, but this rarely leads to the deformities seen in rheumatoid arthritis. Muscle pain and weakness are commonly seen. SLE patients often have various skin rashes. The most characteristic, a "butterfly" rash, appears as a redness appearing over the bridge of the nose and cheeks in the form of a butterfly. Other types of skin rashes appear on almost any part of the body.

Hair loss is quite common in SLE patients.

Raynaud's phenomenon, a disorder in which the blood vessels in the extremities go into spasm on exposure to cold, is also frequent. The hands turn white and pale, eventually blue, and occasionally red. This may lead to ulcerations. Ulcers over the lower extremities are often present.

SLE can affect many different organ systems. In some patients, the linings of the lungs and heart are involved in the disease, leading to pleurisy and pericarditis. If the lungs themselves are affected, the patient may suffer pneumonias and hemorrhage into the lung. Heart problems include heart failure and abnormalities of the coronary arteries.

Kidney damage is a major cause of illness and death, when the disease causes kidney inflammation. This leads to diffuse swelling of the body and eventual kidney failure.

If SLE attacks the nervous system, various types of neurological problems may follow, among them seizures, strokes, psychoses, and various psychiatric and psychological problems.

The gastrointestinal tract may be involved, resulting in weight loss, abdominal pain, gangrene of the bowel, and inability to absorb nutrients.

Because SLE patients often have secondary Sjögren's syndrome, they experience characteristic symptoms of dry eyes and dry mouth. Other SLE patients, however, have no symptoms of dryness and are totally unaware of the presence of SS. Yet when special tests are undertaken, inflammation of these glands is frequently found.

In some patients with connective tissue diseases, biopsies of the inner aspect of the lip may show the same kind of inflammation seen in SS patients. These patients may not have any of the recognizable symptoms.

Unless the patient has SS symptoms, special tests for tear and salivary gland involvement on every patient with SLE or other connective tissue disorder serve no purpose.

Treatment of SLE is very complex and depends on clinical signs and symptoms of the disease. Patients with only a skin rash and joint pain may require nothing more than aspirin and rest over many years.

Patients who have a more progressive type of illness or frequent flare-ups may require steroids (cortisone derivatives), antimalarial medicines, immunosuppressive agents, or other strong drugs, which may decrease the inflammation and stop the progression of the illness. They may also require medicines to control heart failure or high blood pressure, surgical replacement of diseased joints, or kidney dialysis.

POLYMYOSITIS/DERMATOMYOSITIS (PM/DM)

Polymyositis is an acquired (not inherited) disease of the muscles. Patients experience severe weakness in the major voluntary muscles. When accompanied by a characteristic rash, it is called dermatomyositis.

Patients may complain of fatigue, as well as joint and muscle pain, but the major symptom is muscle weakness, usually in the so-called proximal muscles in the areas of the body close to the trunk, that is, in the shoulder and hip girdle.

The patient has difficulty getting up from a chair, walking, getting out of a bathtub, raising the arms to comb the hair, and performing simple tasks. When the disease is more profound, the patient may have no muscle strength at all.

Polymyositis may even involve the muscles of respiration, causing breathing difficulties, and the muscles that control swallowing. PM/DM patients have other symptoms that we normally associate with various connective tissue diseases, including joint pain, joint swelling, and Raynaud's phenomenon, but usually not as prominently as in SLE.

Sometimes, PM/DM may be associated with a malignancy somewhere in the body. Therefore, every PM/DM patient must be examined for a malignancy as part of the medical workup.

The diagnosis of PM/DM is usually based on the typical clinical picture and abnormalities in certain blood tests. These hint to the physician that the muscles are inflamed. Electromyographic (EMG) studies are often performed. The disease is confirmed by a biopsy of involved muscle, which indicates characteristic inflammation. The diagnosis can occasionally be made in the absence of a positive biopsy.

Sjögren's syndrome, both obvious and subtle, can occur in patients with polymyositis.

PM/DM can be very well controlled with corticosteroids and immunosuppressive medicines. Generally, physicians use cortisone derivatives first and immunosuppressive medicines, such as azathioprine and methotrexate, only if the steroids fail or the amount necessary to control the disease causes unsatisfactory side effects. Some physicians are beginning to use immunosuppressives earlier. Because the indications for using immunosuppressive medicines are not uniform among specialists in the field, the treatment of PM/DM is in flux.

Many patients eventually go into spontaneous remission. Death following swallowing difficulty and progressive malnutrition is no longer as frequent as it once was.

When Sjögren's syndrome accompanies polymyositis, it is treated the same way as primary SS. However, SS may respond to an extent to some of the measures used to treat PM/DM.

SCLERODERMA

The most characteristic feature of scleroderma is a thickening and tightening of the skin due to a deposition of excessive amounts of a protein called collagen, normally present in the skin. The reason for the excessive accumulation of collagen is unknown. Changes in the blood vessels and reactions of the immune system are among theories for the cause of this illness.

Similar processes in the internal organs may cause damage to the gastrointestinal, pulmonary, cardiac, and renal systems. Involvement of the esophagus may lead to swallowing difficulties. If the small intestine is affected, patients have difficulty absorbing nutrients, and diarrhea may occur. Involvement of the large bowel may cause constipation. When the lung is affected, the patient may cough and be short of breath. Heart involvement is manifested by shortness of breath and disturbances in the heartbeat. Should the kidneys be affected, rapidly progressive kidney failure and marked high blood pressure may follow. The blood vessels may be inflamed, causing ulcers and gangrene of the extremities.

As many as 95% of scleroderma patients have Raynaud's phenomenon. Joints and muscles are frequently involved, resulting in joint pain, swelling, stiffening, and tightness of the joints. Muscle involvement may result in significant muscle weakness.

The severity of scleroderma, as in most connective tissue diseases, varies. Scleroderma may be an illness with only minimal thickening of one portion of the skin or an illness in which the entire body becomes leatherlike and all organ systems are damaged. When only the skin is affected, patients have a much better outlook than those with systemic sclerosis, the more severe form of the disease.

No one knows what causes scleroderma. Many theories have been proposed. Sjögren's syndrome may complicate scleroderma, as it does RA, SLE, and PM/DM. SS may be obvious and apparent in scleroderma patients who have dry eyes or a dry mouth. In others, it is found only when specifically sought through some of the special tests for SS.

There is no specific treatment for scleroderma. Recent evidence, however, indicates that d-penicillamine, effective in the treatment of RA, may also retard the progression of scleroderma. Generally, treatment is supportive. Pain relievers and anti-inflammatory medicines are used to control joint pain and stiffness. Physiotherapy is very important to maintain range of motion and prevent further contractures. Salves and emollients are used to soften the skin.

When kidney problems and high blood pressure complicate the disease, various antihypertensive medicines, particularly captopril, are quite useful.

Treatment of Sjögren's syndrome itself is similar to the treatment of SS not complicated by scleroderma.

MIXED CONNECTIVE TISSUE DISEASE (MCTD)

In the last few years, doctors have recognized that some patients who have a connective tissue disease do not fall exactly into the categories previously described. Because they manifest some of the features of one or more of the diseases simultaneously, physicians used to see these patients as having overlap syndromes. Others referred to them as patients with mixed connective tissue disease (MCTD).

Besides features normally associated with polymyositis, scleroderma, and SLE, MCTD patients have an antibody to an extractable nuclear antigen (ENA) in their blood, thought to be characteristic of the syndrome. Other physicians believe that patients with so-called MCTD actually have either scleroderma, polymyositis, or SLE. Sjögren's syndrome can also accompany MCTD.

Until we know the specific causes of any of these diseases, further knowledge will be necessary to know whether MCTD is a different entity or one of the other connective tissue diseases.

Treatment depends on primary manifestations. MCTD patients with symptoms of polymyositis often repond to corticosteroids. If primary manifestations are skin tightening or hardening, corticosteroids usually are not very effective.

Treatment of Sjögren's syndrome complicating MCTD is similar to treatment of SS.

WHY SJOGREN'S SYNDROME IS BELIEVED TO BE AN AUTOIMMUNE DISEASE

When Sjögren's syndrome is associated with connective tissue diseases, such as rheumatoid arthritis and systemic lupus erythematosus, an autoimmune process is presumed to underlie the secondary Sjögren's syndrome.

However, physicians often see SS patients who have various features of autoimmune disease, including inflammation of the joints, kidneys, liver, and gastrointestinal tract, who do not fall into any of the strict categories of connective tissue diseases described here. These patients have primary Sjögren's syndrome.

Autoimmunity seems to be very common in these primary SS patients. Clinical evidence hints that the dryness of the eyes and mouth resulting from lymphocyte infiltration into the lacrimal and salivary glands results from an autoimmune process. For example, patients who receive a graft from another individual may develop what is called graft-versus-host disease, in which tissue transplanted to the patient seems to reject the host. These patients often have a disorder that is nearly identical to Sjögren's syndrome as well. This suggests that primary SS is also a result of autoimmunity.

11

Lungs

Daniel M. Libby, M.D.

The upper airway (mouth, throat, and nose), the lower airway (trachea or windpipe) and its branches (the bronchi), and the lungs themselves may be involved in Sjögren's syndrome (SS). Mucous gland dysfunction is the hallmark of SS, and the internal linings of the upper and lower airways and the lungs contain mucous glands. Microscopically, the glands are found to be flooded with lymphocytes (white blood cells), which are thought to cause the dysfunction.

The precise incidence of pulmonary (pertaining to the lungs) involvement in Sjögren's syndrome is uncertain. Estimates range from 1% to 60%. Because pulmonary disorders are commonly seen in association with other autoimmune diseases, such as rheumatoid arthritis, systemic lupus erythematosus, and scleroderma, it is difficult to sort out the forms of pulmonary involvement commonly seen in these diseases from those that are peculiar to SS.

TABLE 1. PULMONARY MANIFESTATIONS OF SJOGREN'S SYNDROME

Upper respiratory tract
  Atrophic rhinitis (nasal dryness)
  Xerostomia (dry mouth)

Lower respiratory tract
  Tracheobronchitis (dryness of the tracheobronchial tree, made up of the trachea and its branches, the bronchi)
  Recurrent infections
  Bronchitis (infection of the bronchial tubes, leading to fever, cough, and sputum)
  Bronchiectasis (weakening of the bronchial tubes, leading to chronic cough and sputum production)
  Acute pneumonia
  Lung abscess (serious lung infection with resultant cavity)

Bronchiolitis* (inflammation of small bronchial tubes)

Atelectasis* (partial collapse of lung segment, often with mucous plugging)

Interstitial pneumonia, chronic* (inflammation and scar tissue in the substance of the lung)

Pleurisy* (inflammation of the pleura, the lungs' lining)

Pulmonary hypertension and vasculitis* (high pressure in the lungs' blood vessels)

Amyloidosis (formation of starchlike substance in the lungs)

Diaphragmatic dysfunction* (disorder of the muscle separating the abdomen and heart and lung cavity)

Pseudolymphoma (an abnormal accumulation of lymphocytes, either in the interstitium of the lung or in lymph glands in the center of the chest)

Malignant lymphoma (cancer of the lymph glands)

---

* disorders found in other collagen vascular disorders

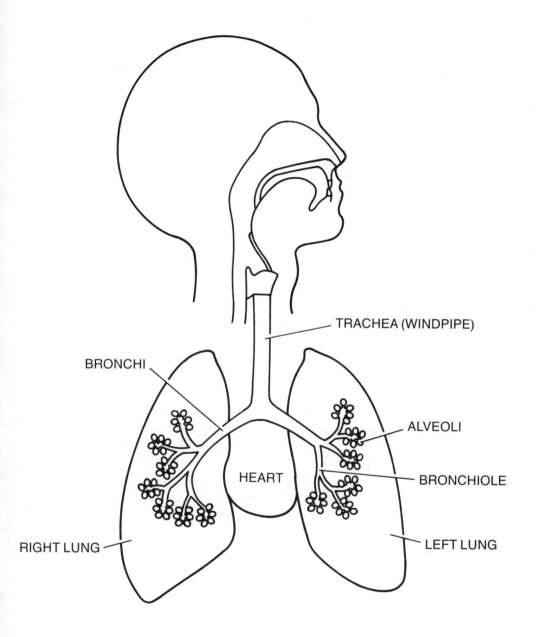

Sites of pulmonary involvement in Sjögren's syndrome.

ASPIRATION PNEUMONIA

Xerostomia (dry mouth) causes pulmonary problems in two ways. First, a dry mouth not only makes swallowing difficult, it causes patients to be unable to soften food well enough to pass it to the back of the throat and into the esophagus. Occasionally, food or liquid goes the wrong way and is aspirated into the lungs. The patient coughs to clear the lungs of the foreign material.

Sometimes, food particles remain in the lung and cause a pneumonia called aspiration pneumonia. The cardinal symptoms are cough, sputum, fever, and in severe cases, shortness of breath. Confirmed by a standard chest x-ray, aspiration pneumonia is treated with antibiotics, usually in the hospital.

ANAEROBIC PNEUMONIA AND LUNG ABSCESS

Because a dry mouth also leads to dental caries and gingival (gum) infection, bacteria from the tooth or gum infection may be passed into the lung, either during sleep or because of ineffective swallowing. This leads to a type of pneumonia often caused by anaerobic bacteria (bacteria that grow best without oxygen). If not properly treated, anaerobic pneumonia commonly leads to a lung abscess.

The patient may have anaerobic pneumonia and lung abscess for weeks or months before it becomes apparent. The symptoms are weight loss, fever, and foul-smelling or foul-tasting sputum.

Anaerobic pneumonia, diagnosed from the patient's history and chest x-ray, requires several weeks of treatment with antibiotics, such as penicillin or clindamycin. Since SS patients have a higher than normal incidence of side effects from antibiotics, particularly certain types of penicillin, drug therapy must be individualized.

ESOPHAGEAL PROBLEMS

Regurgitation of food or drink may be caused by abnormalities of the esophagus in SS patients. These problems, including esophageal hypomotility (loss of the usual muscular contractions in the esophagus that promote food passage from the mouth to the stomach), achalasia (muscular spasm in the lower portion of the esophagus), and webs (bands of tissue blocking the opening of the esophagus) are thoroughly discussed in Chapter 7.

Medication directed at the underlying problem or surgical intervention may be required.

LARYNGOTRACHEOBRONCHITIS

Laryngotracheobronchitis (chronic inflammation of the voice box, windpipe, and bronchial tubes, punctuated by acute infectious episodes) is caused by mucous gland dysfunction in Sjögren's syndrome patients. When mucous production decreases, both in quality (thickness) and in quantity, the SS patient is unable to clear foreign matter that has been inhaled into the respiratory tract. This leads to chronic inflammation of laryngotracheobronchitis.

Cough, the main symptom, can be debilitating. Because of fatigue or malnutrition, mucus becomes inspissated (stuck in the small bronchi), leading to atelectasis (collapse of a segment of lung due to the lack of ventilation to that area). Eventually, pneumonia may result.

TRACHEOBRONCHITIS

Mild tracheobronchitis (inflammation of the windpipe and bronchial tubes) is quite common in Sjögren's syndrome patients. Some studies have suggested an incidence up to 50%. Symptoms include chest burning, pain associated with breathing, shortness of breath, wheezing, and hoarseness of voice.

In contrast to its usefulness in diagnosing pneumonia, a standard chest x-ray is usually normal and not helpful in diagnosing tracheobronchitis. Results of pulmonary function tests are more sensitive in supporting the patient's history. Although there are many types of breathing tests, the diagnosis of tracheobronchitis may be confirmed from simple spirometry. In this test, which may be performed in the doctor's office, the patient is asked to take a

deep breath, then exhale into a tube as rapidly as possible, repeat
ing this several times. In tracheobronchitis, vital capacity (total
amount of air exhaled) may be normal, but the rate at which it is
exhaled is slow. This indicates an obstructive ventilatory impairment or blockage of air flow.

RELIEF TREATMENTS FOR TRACHEOBRONCHITIS

Humidifying mists from properly cleaned room humidifiers
or medically prescribed nebulizers may be helpful. Nebulizers
break up water droplets into fine microscopic particles, freely sus-
pended in the air, and thus capable of reaching the smallest bronchioles.

If the patient is wheezing or if a blockage to air flow is found
on pulmonary function tests, then bronchodilator medications
may be prescribed. These medications, which come in tablet, capsule, or aerosol mist form, relax the smooth muscle surrounding
the bronchial tubes, partially relieving the blockage.

Bronchodilators are used to treat this condition, but this must
be done with caution, especially in persons with cardiovascular
diseases. Occasional side effects include palpitations (rapid or irregular heartbeat), tremor, insomnia, anxiety, and gastrointestinal
upsets, such as nausea, vomiting, and diarrhea.

Numerous types of methyl xanthines are given orally or in-
travenously. If bronchodilators and methyl xanthines are not helpful, the physician may try corticosteroids, such as prednisone, Me-
drol, or cortisone. Corticosteroids have both anti-inflammatory
and bronchodilator properties. In many cases, they destroy the
abnormal accumulation of lymphocytes in the mucous glands of
the tracheobronchial tree and are successful in treating tracheobronchitis in Sjögren's syndrome patients.

Corticosteroids may have serious side effects, if taken at high
doses or for prolonged periods. They must be taken under close
medical supervision for only severe manifestations of SS, whether
pulmonary or for symptoms in other parts of the body.

BRONCHIOLITIS

Bronchiolitis (inflammation of bronchial tube branches less than 2 mm. in diameter) has been recognized only recently as a problem for Sjögren's syndrome patients. As a consequence of accumulated lymphocytes in the mucous glands, bronchioles may become permanently obstructed by mucus or scar tissue.

Once believed to be rare, bronchiolitis is now thought to be fairly common in Sjögren's syndrome. In one study, the disorder was found in six of 13 SS patients, but was serious in only two. Although the prognosis for broncholitis is usually poor, it may improve, if the disease is recognized and treated earlier.

As in tracheobronchitis, pulmonary function tests, chiefly spirometry, are most helpful in making the diagnosis. Chest x-rays are less useful.

INTERSTITIAL PNEUMONIA

As the bronchi successively branch into bronchioles, they end in microscopic-size air sacs called alveoli. The millions of alveoli in the lungs are embedded in supporting tissue known as the interstitium. Within the interstitium are capillaries (tiny blood vessels) that take oxygen from and give carbon dioxide to the alveoli.

In interstitial pneumonia, an abnormal accumulation of lymphocytes and scar tissue in the supporting tissue around the alveoli form a barrier to the speedy exchange of oxygen and carbon dioxide between the alveoli and the capillaries. As blood oxygen content drops, organs throughout the body may malfunction. The patient complains of shortness of breath on exertion. As the lungs become abnormally stiff, the patient develops a rapid shallow breathing pattern. Although cough is a common symptom, sputum production is less likely. Chest x-ray and pulmonary function tests are abnormal. Pulmonary function tests measure a reduced volume of air in the lungs, while the rate of air entry and exit is normal or supernormal.

An additional pulmonary function test for early indications of interstitial pneumonia in Sjögren's syndrome is the diffusing capacity test, which measures the rate of gas transfer from the air sacs to the lungs' blood vessels. This test may be done in a pulmonary specialist's office or in a hospital pulmonary function laboratory.

The severity of interstitial pneumonia may vary from no symptoms to a disabling shortness of breath at rest. Lymphocytic interstitial pneumonia (LIP), a form of interstitial pneumonia peculiar to SS, is usually treated with corticosteroids. It does not cause long-term disability. If not treated early, interstitial pneumonia may progress to an end stage and may be untreatable.

INTERSTITIAL PNEUMONITIS

The distinction between interstitial pneumonia and interstitial pneumonitis (inflammation of the supporting tissue around the alveoli of the lungs) is subtle. A recent study suggests that many Sjögren's syndrome patients may have interstitial pneumonitis long before symptoms appear or before the chest x-ray and pulmonary function tests become abnormal.

The study used a new technique, the gallium scan, to detect inflammation in the lung. The patient is given an injection of gallium, a radioisotope, which is taken up in areas of inflammation throughout the body. After 48 to 72 hours, lung inflammation will show up on a scan of the lungs.

Interstitial pneumonitis is treated with corticosteroids, when there is evidence of a clearcut deterioration in lung function. The Sjögren's syndrome patient is given a trial of corticosteroids and reassessed at the end of four to six weeks. If the patient has a good response, the dose is slowly lowered and the patient closely monitored for possible relapse. If the patient has not improved after six weeks, corticosteroids should be discontinued, because the risk of harmful side effects begins to outweigh the possible benefits.

DISTINGUISHING INTERSTITIAL PNEUMONITIS FROM OTHER CONDITIONS

Interstitial pneumonitis in Sjögren's syndrome patients needs to be differentiated from infection, pseudolymphoma (an abnormally high accumulation of lymphocytes in the lungs or lymph glands of the chest), lymphoma (cancer of the lymph glands), and other conditions. Therefore, a lung biopsy is often needed.

A lung biopsy is performed either through a chest incision (open lung biopsy) under general anesthesia or through a flexible bronchoscope, a narrow tube that enables the physician to see into the bronchial tubes. While the patient is awake under local anesthesia, the bronchoscope is passed through the nose. Biopsies taken in bronchoscopy are satisfactory for excluding infection, but may not provide a large or representative enough sample to distinguish between inflammatory or tumorous conditions. In these cases, an open lung biopsy may be advisable.

PLEURISY

Pleurisy (inflammation of the lining around the lungs) usually causes chest or shoulder pain on breathing. Pleural effusion (fluid accumulation in the pleural space) may lead to shortness of breath.

Pleurisy is treated with corticosteroids, as well as nonsteroidal anti-inflammatory drugs. In some cases, drainage of fluid may be necessary.

PULMONARY HYPERTENSION

Pulmonary hypertension is an abnormally high pressure in the pulmonary arteries, the blood vessels carrying blood from the heart to the lungs. Drugs designed to dilate pulmonary arteries are used, such as nitroglycerine, nifedipine (Procardia), and hydralazine.

PULMONARY PSEUDOLYMPHOMA

Pulmonary pseudolymphoma is an abnormal accumulation of lymphocytes, either in the interstitium of the lung or in the lymph glands in mediastinum, the center of the chest. Microscopically and on x-ray, pseudolymphoma may resemble lymphoma or lymphosarcoma, a malignant tumor of the lymph glands.

Pseudolymphoma may be asymptomatic, appearing only on a routine x-ray. Or, by putting pressure on nearby lung structures, it may cause chest pain, cough, wheezing, or shortness of breath.

To make the diagnosis, a lymph node or a lung biopsy is necessary. The slides should be reviewed by a pathologist experienced in differentiating the benign pseudolymphoma from malignant lymphoma. This distinction is often difficult, and experts may disagree. The prognosis for pseudolymphoma is good. It may improve without treatment or may need treatment with corticosteroids. In a very few cases, pseudolymphoma develops into a malignant lymphoma.

MALIGNANT LYMPHOMA

Malignant lymphoma (cancer of the lymph glands) develops in a very small percentage (less than 5%) of Sjögren's syndrome patients, more commonly in those who do not have an associated collagen vascular disorder.

It may affect any organ in the body, commonly causing fever, weight loss, anemia, night sweats, and itching of the skin. Pulmonary symptoms are similar to pseudolymphoma.

A lymph node biopsy must be performed to make the diagnosis. Treatment may include radiation therapy (cobalt) and/or chemotherapy, with or without corticosteroids. The prognosis is variable.

12

Kidneys

Stuart S. Kassan, M.D.
Robert J. Kassan, M.D.

Long recognized as a complex condition responsible for dryness of the eyes, nose, and mouth, Sjögren's syndrome (SS) also involves extraglandular organs and systems. Not the least of these is the renal or kidney system.

Kidney conditions can occur in both primary Sjögren's syndrome, in which the sicca (dryness) complex is not associated with an underlying disease, and in secondary SS, in which the patient has an associated connective tissue disorder, particularly rheumatoid arthritis or systemic lupus erythematosus.

In either case, the basic problem is similar. Something has gone wrong with the immune system, the body's defense against disease. An overproduction of white blood cells, called lymphocytes, invade body tissues, interfering with normal functions, such as the production of tears and saliva. The lymphocytes produce unusual proteins, called autoantibodies, which may also lead to organ malfunction.

A similar process occurs when the kidneys are affected in Sjögren's syndrome. Immune elements, including lymphocytes, antibodies, cryoglobulins (a form of protein in the blood), and an unusual macroglobulin (large protein) are deposited in the kidney tissues. In some puzzling instances, the exact location and extent can be determined by means of a kidney biopsy.

MANIFESTATIONS OF KIDNEY DISEASE

Kidney diseases in Sjögren's syndrome are of several types, depending on which element of the renal system is involved. A thorough study and complete history of the patient is important.

The most common kidney condition seen in SS patients is *interstitial nephritis.* Because this causes difficulty in producing a concentrated urine, patients with interstitial nephritis urinate more frequently and in larger quantities.

Sjögren's syndrome patients may have a condition known as *renal tubular acidosis,* in which the patient is unable to excrete a highly acid urine. This may cause a severe depletion of potassium in the blood, resulting in an electrolyte imbalance, a condition in which the amounts of normal essential blood chemicals—such as sodium, chloride, carbon dioxide, calcium, phosphorus, and urea nitrogen, as well as potassium—are changed. These alterations can result in the impairment of important physiological functions, including heart action, muscle contraction, and nerve conduction. A further important consideration is the possible lowering of the pH value in the blood, which is normally maintained with little room for variation. The lowering of the pH value, indicating an acidity reaction, will result in an acidosis.

In many instances, renal tubular acidosis has no obvious clinical symptoms, so the condition is unrecognized. At other times, kidney symptoms may appear before the sicca symptoms. Other findings include calcification of the kidney, kidney stones, and a lower urinary citrate concentration.

Occasionally, a Sjögren's syndrome patient will have a true *glomerulonephritis,* an inflammation of the glomerulus or filtering element of the kidney. This is brought about because the immune complex has been deposited only in this part of the kidney. One group of investigators noted an associated purpura (areas of bleeding in the skin), hematuria (blood in the urine), proteinuria (albumin in the urine), and marked hypertension. These patients also had high levels of rheumatoid factor (RF) and moderate levels of antinuclear antibodies (ANAs), both of which are signs of a underlying connective tissue disease. These patients are assumed to have secondary SS.

DIAGNOSTIC TESTS

Whenever a patient has a definite or suspected case of Sjögren's syndrome, the investigation of all systems, including the renal system, must be thorough, because of the wide range of possible disorders in addition to kidney and glandular disorders. Some of these problems are latent, often having no symptoms for long periods of time.

Whenever the physician suspects the possibility of Sjögren's syndrome, a complete study of the kidney must be conducted. This study should include measurements of electrolytes (blood sodium, potassium, chloride, and bicarbonate), as well as blood urea nitrogen and serum creatinine. In addition, the urine should be studied for albumin and a determination of the reaction (pH value). A 24-hour urine test for creatinine clearance should be completed.

If the patient has had kidney symptoms for a long time, an intravenous pyelogram (IVP), a kidney x-ray taken after an opaque dye has been injected into the bloodstream, may be required to determine the possible presence of calcium deposits.

In rare instances, when there is a marked degree of kidney impairment, a kidney biopsy may be necessary.

TREATMENTS

There is no specific treatment for kidney involvement in Sjögren's syndrome. In many instances, particularly in interstitial nephritis and renal tubular acidosis, the abnormalities are latent and require no treatment. However, regular follow-up is strongly suggested.

With more overt manifestations of disease, specifically kidney stones, calcification of the kidney, and elevated urinary pH values, alkaline agents are used to prevent or reverse the potential development of metabolic acidosis (lowered pH values) and to prevent lowered potassium values.

In some cases, when progressive renal insufficiency develops and specifically when renal function worsens, a kidney biopsy may be done. Depending on the findings, corticosteroid (cortisone) therapy may be used. In more severe situations, immunosuppresive therapy (chemotherapy) may be needed.

The most common adverse reactions to immunosuppressive therapy include mouth ulcers, leukopenia (lowered white blood cell count), nausea, and abdominal distress. In addition, there can be chills and fever, loss of hair, skin rashes, bone marrow depression, and kidney involvement, resulting in failing function. In view of the potentially serious and sometimes life-threatening reactions that may result from immunosuppresive drugs, their use must be considered as a calculated risk.

CONCLUSION

Kidney involvement in Sjögren's syndrome is not uncommon. However, the percentage of patients with overt clinical manifestations is not significant. Many cases can be determined only by specific tests. When there is evidence of progressive deterioration of kidney function, frequent observations and appropriate tests should be performed. Depending on the findings, aggressive therapy should be pursued in an attempt to control the progress of failing kidney function.

Because of the manifold accompanying manifestations of kidney involvement in Sjögrens' syndrome, nothing takes the place of a periodic history, physical examination, and frequent follow-up to detect some of these abnormalities.

13

Blood Vessels

Andrew P. Andonopoulos, M.D.
Haralampos M. Moutsopoulos, M.D.

A variety of illnesses characterized by inflammation and eventual destruction of the blood vessel wall are included under the umbrella term *vasculitis*. In general, vasculitis is a feature of all connective tissue diseases. As such, it can complicate primary Sjögren's syndrome (SS).

A classification of the various disorders known as vasculitis appears at the end of this chapter.

FACTORS INVOLVED IN THE PROCESS OF VASCULITIS

Two biologic processes are operating in the development of the vessel wall injury. First, immune complexes (aggregates or clusters of antigens and their antibodies) are deposited on the vessel wall. These deposits successively activate a series of immunologically important blood proteins, called complement components, and induce inflammation and tissue destruction. Second, activated lymphocytes (cells of the body's defense system) destroy the vessel wall.

During the inflammatory and subsequent healing process, narrowing and closing of the inside of the blood vessel result in ischemia (decreased blood supply) of the organs and tissues whose vessels are affected by the vasculitis. This is manifested by the impaired function of the particular organs. The injury can progress to necrosis (tissue death).

WHICH SJOGREN'S SYNDROME PATIENTS DEVELOP VASCULITIS?

The clinical experience of physicians treating Sjögren's syndrome patients suggests that vasculitis usually occurs several years after the diagnosis of primary SS has been established.

Furthermore, primary Sjögren's syndrome patients affected by vasculitis are mainly those with more widespread extraglandular disease. As a rule, vasculitis complicates SS that is not confined to the exocrine glands, that is, SS that is not limited to such manifestations as dry eyes and dry mouth. Vasculitis usually occurs in patients with Raynaud's phenomenon (sequential change in finger color from white to blue to red, occurring with minimal environmental temperature fall or with psychological stress); enlarged lymph nodes, liver, and spleen; kidney and lung involvement; and commonly detected serum cryoglobulins (specific protein complexes circulating in the blood that are deposited during cold).

WHAT BLOOD VESSELS ARE INVOLVED AND WHAT IS THE CLINICAL PICTURE OF SJOGREN'S SYNDROME VASCULITIS?

The types of vessels affected by vasculitis in Sjögren's syndrome patients include:
- small vessels (arterioles, capillaries, and venules), which represent the very minute terminal branches of arteries and veins
- medium-size arteries, for example, those that supply the bowel

Skin is the most commonly affected organ. Inflammation and destruction of capillaries and venules, with subsequent blood leakage, are responsible for the appearance of the skin. The Sjögren's syndrome patient with skin vasculitis usually presents with a *purpura*, a condition characterized by hemorrhage into the skin. In SS, it appears as crops of petechiae (very small, red spots, the size of a pin or a little larger). These may be itchy, usually can be felt, and are located mainly in the lower extremities and buttocks. The lesions come and go, do not blanch under pressure, and may leave a residual brownish discoloration at the site after the red spots disappear.

The next most common presenting symptom of vasculitis in Sjögren's syndrome patients is *urticaria* (hives), which may or may not contain petechiae and usually do not itch.

Other, less commonly observed skin lesions include *erythema multiforme* (larger red spots with a pale center); *erythema nodosum* (red, hot, tender lesions of various sizes, involving the skin and the underlying fatty tissue); or *skin ulcers* in the lower legs.

Should the arteries supplying the fingers and toes be affected, a violet discoloration appears in these areas, which can progress to *gangrene* (tissue death) of the terminal part of a finger or a toe.

Vasculitis of the small vessels supplying the nerves with blood results in *peripheral neuropathy*. This is expressed by numbness, tingling, pains, loss of sensation, and weakness in both hands and feet symmetrically in a so-called "glove-and-stocking" distribution. Sometimes, a more serious problem occurs, called *mononeuritis multiplex*, meaning paralysis of one or more major nerve branches. This results in foot drop or hand drop.

A *myositis* (muscle inflammation), usually mild and manifested as diffuse muscle pains, is rather common in Sjögren's syndrome. This is caused by a mild vasculitis involving the blood vessels of the muscles.

Very rarely, a vasculitis of medium-size arteries may produce serious problems in Sjögren's syndrome patients. When the arteries supplying such organs as the small or large bowel or gallbladder are closed, the subsequent decrease in blood supply to such organs can lead to necrosis and perforation, resulting in *peritonitis* (inflammation of the abdominal cavity). This can be fatal, if not treated promptly with surgery.

Involvement of the small and medium-size arteries supplying the kidneys leads to glomerular inflammation, producing what we call *glomerulonephritis*. This is expressed clinically by peripheral edema (swelling), high blood pressure, and abnormal urine analysis.

HOW DO PHYSICIANS DIAGNOSE VASCULITIS IN SJOGREN'S SYNDROME PATIENTS?

The first clue to the diagnosis of vasculitis in Sjögren's syndrome patients is the clinical presentation, that is, the symptoms that prompted the patient to seek medical attention.

Angiography (x-rays taken after a radio-opaque dye is injected into the artery) does not play as large a role in the diagnostic workup of SS patients with vasculitis as it does in polyarteritis nodosa patients, in whom it may reveal characteristic micro-aneurysms (small sacs of the arterial wall).

The diagnosis of vasculitis in Sjögren's syndrome patients is confirmed by biopsy. If the skin is involved, biopsy of an area with lesions will disclose the characteristic picture of small vessel vasculitis. Muscle biopsy may reveal a similar inflammation in the vessels supplying the muscle with blood. In cases of neuropathy, biopsy of a sural nerve (a small nerve branch in the calf of the leg) will confirm the diagnosis.

Additional laboratory abnormalities observed in SS patients with vasculitis include a high erythrocyte (red blood cell) sedimentation rate, anemia (below normal level of red blood cells), and the detection of hypergammaglobulinemia (elevation of a portion of blood proteins called gamma globulins), cryoglobulins in the serum, low complement levels (indicating their consumption in the inflammatory process), and high titers of specific autoantibodies (antibodies against self), such as rheumatoid factor (RF) and antinuclear antibodies (ANAs). Figures of these laboratory abnormalities, obtained from a recent study, appear in the following table.

PREVALENCE OF LABORATORY ABNORMALITIES IN NINE PRIMARY SJOGREN'S SYNDROME PATIENTS WITH VASCULITIS

Laboratory abnormality	Number of patients
Increased gamma globulins	7
Positive rheumatoid factor	9
Positive antinuclear antibodies	9
Cryoglobulins in serum	9
Low serum complement	7

WHAT DO PHYSICIANS DO FOR VASCULITIS IN SJOGREN'S SYNDROME AND WHAT IS THE PROGNOSIS?

If skin involvement is the only manifestation of vasculitis in a Sjögren's syndrome patient, this condition is benign and specific measures are not necessary. The physician usually recommends only that the patient keep his or her legs elevated, to avoid the aggravating effect of gravity on the development of petechiae (red spots).

The term "benign" could, with some reservations, be applied to most other manifestations of vasculitis in Sjögren's syndrome patients. This is because SS patients with vasculitis usually respond well to appropriate treatment, better than do patients with other forms of idiopathic (of unknown cause) vasculitis. In SS patients whose muscles, kidneys, or nerves are affected by vasculitis, such drugs as corticosteroids and cyclophosphamide (a medication that suppresses the immune response, which is given either by mouth or by intermittent intravenous injections) are necessary and the results are beneficial.

Sometimes, especially when the serious manifestations noted above are related to cryoglobulins circulating in the blood, the physician will recommend plasmapheresis, a technique in which the patient's blood is removed by a machine similar to a dialysis machine and cleansed of circulating immune complexes and cryo-globulins.

Finally, in a patient in whom vasculitis causes perforation of an abdominal organ and peritonitis, the prognosis depends on the promptness of surgical intervention.

CONCLUSION

Early recognition of vasculitis in Sjögren's syndrome patients and appropriate medical intervention give these patients the promise of a beneficial outcome.

CLASSIFICATION OF VASCULITIS

In their attempts to classify disorders known as vasculitis, experts in the field consider such important factors as the size of the involved vessels (small, medium, large); the lesion identified by the pathologist by looking at the injured vessel under the microscope; and the successive biological events leading to the observed damage. However, a completely satisfactory classification has not appeared so far, mainly because of our inability to identify specific causes of most of these maladies.

One of the most successful classifications is that proposed by researcher Anthony S. Fauci, M.D., and his co-workers, in which the following kinds of vasculitis are recognized: polyarteritis nodosa, hypersensitivity vasculitis, Wegener's granulomatosis, giant cell arteritis, Takayasu's arteritis, Kawasaki's disease, and Buerger's disease.

The following are brief descriptions and hallmarks of the above entities:

Polyarteritis nodosa group: This includes the classic polyarteritis nodosa, the allergic granulomatosis (Churg-Strauss disease), and overlap syndromes. Medium-size muscular arteries, arterioles, and venules are affected by inflammation. Almost every organ, including kidneys, intestinal tract and liver, central and peripheral nervous systems, heart, muscles, and joints can be involved. Almost one-third of patients with polyarteritis are hepatitis B antigen-positive. Due to involvement of vital organs, the disease is serious, but prognosis has improved considerably with the use of cyclophosphamide, a cytotoxic drug.

Hypersensitivity vasculitis: A heterogeneous group of disorders thought to represent a hypersensitivity reaction, usually to a drug or an infectious agent. Small vessels, including arterioles and venules (the very small branches of the arteries and veins), are involved. Most frequently the skin is the only organ affected, presenting with palpable purpura or urticaria. Even if other organs are involved, this involvement tends to be less severe than that observed in other systemic types of vasculitis, and still the skin disease remains the dominant feature.

Wegener's granulomatosis: A systemic small vessel vasculitis characterized by involvement of the upper and lower respiratory tracts and kidneys. Variable degrees of other multiple organ involvement (skin, heart, eyes, nervous system, and others) are also characteristic. The disease was once universally fatal, but with cyclophosphamide, the prognosis now is quite good.

Giant cell arteritis: A disease of the elderly, affecting large arteries and their branches. Also called temporal arteritis, it classically causes severe temporal headache due to inflammation of that artery. Biopsy of this artery is essential for the diagnosis of the disease. The most dreaded complication of the disease is sudden, unilateral blindness due to occlusion of the terminal branches of the eye artery. This is irreversible. Corticosteroids are the treatment of choice and usually provide excellent results.

Takayasu's arteritis: An inflammatory disease of the aorta (the main artery originating from the heart) and its branches, affecting mainly young females in Japan. However, increasing numbers are being recognized recently in the United States. Symptoms originate from decreased blood supply to various organs, including the heart and brain, and to the extremities. Corticosteroids are of benefit.

Kawasaki's disease: This is an acute, febrile illness of infants and young children that has occurred in Japan in epidemics, but is described in the United States as well. Patients present with characteristic skin and mucous membrane changes and enlargement of lymph nodes. The disease is self-limited and generally benign, but 1-2% of affected children die from coronary arteritis (vasculitis involving the arteries supplying blood to the heart). Aspirin is the recommended treatment.

Buerger's disease (Thromboangiitis obliterans): Obstructive vascular disease of unknown cause, strongly associated with cigarette smoking, affecting primarily young males. Medium and small arteries and veins of the limbs are involved with inflammation, clotting, and obstruction. Patients have symptoms due to decreased arterial blood supply and may end up with amputation of the extremities. Thrombophlebitis (clot formation in veins) is also common.

SUGGESTED PROFESSIONAL BIBLIOGRAPHY

Fauci AS, *Vasculitis in Clinical Immunology*. CW Parker (ed). Philadelphia: Saunders, pp. 475-519 (1980).

Talal N, Moutsopoulos HM, Kassan, SS (eds), *Sjögren's Syndrome: Clinical and Immunological Aspects*. Berlin, Heidelberg: Springer-Verlag, 1987.

Moutsopoulos HM, Chused TM, Mann DL, Klippel JH, Fauci AS, Frank MM, Lawley TJ, Hamburger MI. Sjögren's syndrome (sicca syndrome): Current issues. *Ann Intern Med* 92: 212-226 (1980).

Tsokos M, Lazarou S, Moutsopoulos HM. Vasculitis in primary Sjögren's syndrome: Histologic classification and clinical presentation. *Amer J Clin Pathol* 88:26-31 (1986).

14

Nervous System

David A. Isenberg, M.D.
Michael L. Snaith, M.D.

As other chapters in this handbook make clear, Sjögren's syndrome (SS) may involve not only dry eyes and dry mouth. In this chapter, some of the ways in which the nervous system can be affected by SS will be reviewed. The recent description by a group of Baltimore physicians of possible multiple sclerosislike symptoms will also be discussed.

The nervous system can be divided into central and peripheral parts. The *central nervous system* incorporates (1) the brain; (2) the so-called cranial nerves, which come directly from the brain and are responsible hearing, seeing, smelling, taste, and other functions; and (3) the spinal cord. The *peripheral nervous system* is the system of nerves passing from the spinal cord throughout the rest of the body.

NEUROLOGICAL MANIFESTATIONS OF SS

In the experience of many neurologists, three common neurological complications of Sjögren's syndrome are: carpal tunnel syndrome, trigeminal neuralgia, and peripheral sensory neuropathy.

Carpal tunnel syndrome, the commonest complication, results from pressure on a special tunnel between the wrist and the palm of the hand called the carpal tunnel, through which the median nerve passes. Typically, this pressure gives rise to feelings of numbness and "pins and needles" in the thumb, first, and second fingers. Some pain may be associated with this. In some patients, the pain seems to spread up the arm towards the elbow. The symptoms are often worse at night.

In contrast, *trigeminal neuralgia* is an electric shock sensation involving the fifth cranial nerve, the nerve providing normal sensation to the face from the cheekbone to the jaw. The pain lasts only a matter of seconds. It might be brought on by movements of the face and jaw, by touching the skin, or by drafts of cold air on the face. Eating and speaking may become extremely difficult. "Trigger spots" on the skin of the face or within the mouth may provoke pain when touched. The acute pain may be followed by another, "boring" type of pain. The attacks are uncommon at night.

Another neurological complication in Sjögren's syndrome is known as *peripheral sensory neuropathy* or *neuritis*. Patients with this condition become aware that their hands and sometimes their feet do not feel normal. Sharp objects do not feel as sharp or cold things as cold. Patients may be able to identify a dividing line or a "level" around their limbs. Below this level, the feeling is abnormal.

Of greater concern, over the past three years, are reports from a group of physicians at Johns Hopkins University in Baltimore describing a serious form of Sjögren's syndrome affecting both the central and peripheral nervous systems, sometimes with psychiatric features. This group has suggested that the more serious neurological problems resemble other well known neurological conditions, such as multiple sclerosis (MS). In the experience of many physicians in the United States and Europe who have discussed these observations, this type of neurological involvement in SS is thought to be very rare.

DIAGNOSTIC TESTS

A careful history and clinical examination usually enable the physician to diagnose carpal tunnel syndrome, trigeminal neuralgia, or peripheral sensory neuropathy with ease. In carpal tunnel syndrome and peripheral neuropathy, certain electrical tests, called nerve conduction studies, measure the speed and amplitude of the electric current in the peripheral nerves and help confirm the diagnosis. These tests involve electrical stimulation of nerves in the arms or legs. The speed of the impulses is recorded by devices attached to the arm or leg, which are some distance from the electric pulse.

Although there is no definitive test for trigeminal neuralgia, it can be recognized clinically.

If a Sjögren's syndrome patient develops a more complicated neurological problem, more sophisticated ways of examining brain function are used. These tests can include the electroencephalogram (EEG), in which a number of recording wires are attached around the head to monitor the brain waves produced constantly in the skull.

In addition, computerized axial tomography (CAT scanning) and the more recently introduced nuclear magnetic resonance (MRI) are widely available to detect structural abnormalities within the brain.

These techniques are noninvasive and require approximately 30 minutes to perform. In sequences of pictures, these scans give a remarkably accurate impression of the structures within the skull. However, they do need to be interpreted by specialists.

TREATMENTS

Carpal tunnel syndrome, trigeminal neuralgia, and peripheral neuropathy are all capable of disappearing spontaneously. These conditions certainly fluctuate from one month to the next. If these problems persist, and certainly, if they seem to be getting worse, it is sensible to describe them in detail to one's physician. After a physicial examination, the physician will organize the appropriate tests and will probably be able to prescribe treatments that will relieve the symptoms.

Carpal tunnel syndrome will respond to diuretic (water-losing) tablets, local corticosteroid injections, or if all else fails, to surgery. Corticosteroid injections may be repeated on two or even more occasions. Relief is transitory, rarely permanent. Surgery usually involves making a small incision on the palmar side of the wrist joint and freeing the tissues that have enmeshed the nerve. In many medical centers, surgery is available on an outpatient basis. Although the postoperative period is a little uncomfortable, the operation is usually very successful.

Trigeminal neuralgia is usually treated by a drug called carbamazepine. Initially introduced to treat epilepsy, this drug has found considerable utility in treating the rather unpleasant symptoms of trigeminal neuralgia. In a high proportion of patients, neurologic symptoms can be abolished by taking these tablets (usually 200 mg. tablets are prescribed) three to five times a day. Unsteadiness and drowsiness are occasional side effects of high doses, but skin rashes and bone marrow effects are extremely rare.

Peripheral neuropathy may prove more difficult to treat. Sometimes, it may be better to wait and see if it remits spontaneously. If not, corticosteroid treatment may be required to help relieve the symptoms.

MORE SERIOUS COMPLICATIONS

Sjögren's syndrome patients should not unnecessarily fear unlikely complications. Anxiety itself is a potentially damaging symptom.

One major problem is that nobody yet has shown that Sjögren's syndrome is a single disease with a single cause. It is quite possible that patients who have SS in association with rheumatoid arthritis, for example, may have a mild process affecting their saliva or tears, but have no risk whatsoever of severe neurological disease.

It is important that physicians consider the possibility of Sjögren's syndrome as a cause for neurological syndromes of various kinds. However, there is a danger that patients who know their dry mouths and dry eyes are due to SS will become worried unnecessarily that they could at any moment develop much more alarming disorders.

In a recent review of over 100 Sjögren's syndrome patients, approximately half had primary SS, with no evidence of another underlying immune disorder; about half had secondary SS, which was secondary to another connective tissue disease, usually systemic lupus erythematosus.

Considering these patients together, about one in six had evidence of neurological problems, virtually all being carpal tunnel syndrome, trigeminal neuralgia, or peripheral sensory neuropathy. Some of these patients have been followed up for as long as 10 years, with no sign of any more sinister neurological complication.

Thus, neurological complications of Sjögren's syndrome, while they clearly exist, are generally considered to be of a fairly mild nature, relatively easy to investigate, and often respond to conventional treatment.

15

Allergy

Paul B. Lang, M.D.

The patient who is eventually diagnosed as having Sjögren's syndrome (SS) often appears first in an allergist's office. This is not surprising, since many of the symptoms of SS initially resemble those of allergic reactions. Red, irritated eyes, dry mouth, sore throat, and stuffy ears and nose, all unexplained by infection, may make one suspicious of allergies. Moreover, during winter months, the symptoms get worse with exposure to dry heating.

Since as many as 10% of the general population have allergies, a patient can have both Sjögren's syndrome and allergies. When working up a patient with SS, however, the allergist may find no association between the symptoms and possible exposure to or ingestion of an allergenic substance. SS patients usually do not complain of sneezing or of itchy eyes and nose. Because of their drying side effects, antihistamines may well have made the SS patient's symptoms worse.

Skin tests for allergies to foods or inhalants will be negative in the patient with Sjögren's syndrome. A blood test for the presence of immunoglobin E, a blood protein that is usually elevated in allergic people, will be within normal limits. Even if allergies are found, an antinuclear antibody (ANA) test should be be ordered for any patient who has symptoms of SS.

When allergies coexist with Sjögren's syndrome, treatment is fraught with much difficulty. The medication best used for one disorder may be contraindicated in the other. Close interaction between the various treating physicians is mandatory.

WHAT CAUSES ALLERGIES?

Allergic people are normal in all ways, except for the over-production of a blood protein called immunoglobin E (IgE). This can be measured by a sensitive blood test. A measurement of over 50 units (depending on the laboratory used) indicates an increased susceptibility to allergic disease.

The symptoms of allergy result from the release of certain chemicals, for example, *histamine,* within the body. These chemicals are stored in cells, called *basophils* and *mast cells,* found even in those who are not allergic.

In allergic individuals, proteins found in foods or the environment, called *allergens,* cause allergic reactions.

ALLERGIC REACTIONS

An allergic reaction occurs when all three components—mast cells, IgE, and an allergen—are present at the same time. Allergic reactions may manifest themselves as skin rashes; wheezing from the chest; itchy, stuffy nose and ears; postnasal drip; or itching and irritated eyes. This can be a seasonal problem, if an individual is allergic to environmental allergens, such as trees, grass, molds, or weeds, or a perennial problem, if the allergen is dust, animals, or foods.

AVOIDING EXPOSURE TO ALLERGENS

The mainstay of allergic treatment is avoiding exposure to known allergens. If a person is allergic to animals, for example, he or she should avoid animals completely or stay away from them as much as possible. Very often, just removing the animal from the bedroom will lessen symptoms.

It is possible to be allergic to one breed of animal and not another. For instance, an allergic reaction to a German shepherd in one person's house may not happen in another house with a Doberman pinscher. One could be allergic to a horse and not other animals. Because all dogs produce dander (dandruff), a major allergen, there is no such thing as a dog that cannot produce allergies in those who are susceptible.

To avoid exposure to animal allergens, one must avoid objects consisting of animal substances, such as mattresses made of hog or horse hair; pillows, comforters, and furniture containing feathers; and carpet linings consisting of cow's hair.

To reduce house dust, a major allergen, the basic room to keep clean is the bedroom, where one ordinarily spends a good deal of time. To facilitate cleaning, the bedroom should be kept as simple as possible, with wood floors, no curtains, little stuffed furniture, and few books and toys. Cleaning daily with a vacuum cleaner, which will remove the dust, is better than shuffling the dust around the room with a cloth.

House mites, microscopic bugs that are a major component of dust, live off human skin. They are, therefore, found in bedding areas. Special mattress and pillow covers that prevent mites from accumulating in bedding are available.

Molds, consisting of microscopic organisms that tend to grow in damp and poorly lit areas, are another source of allergic exposure. Molds are the blackish-greenish material often found on shower curtains or in damp basements. Individuals whose allergies are exacerbated on damp days are often allergic to molds. Once present, molds are hard to eradicate. Cleaning with antifungal agents, Lysol, or ammonia help to destroy the mold.

But the key to removing mold is changing the environment by increasing aeration of the area, by opening windows or doors, or by removing the dampness with a dehumidifier or by sealing leaks. Chemicals are often added to wallpaper paste to prevent mold buildup behind wallpaper.

Perfume, smoke, chemicals, dry air, and other environmental irritants that exacerbate allergic symptoms should be avoided by patients with either Sjögren's syndrome or allergic disease. In some individuals, symptoms worsen with acute changes in barometric pressure or temperature. Knowing that these physical factors can make things worse helps allergic individuals to reduce their symptoms by avoiding exposure.

TESTING FOR ALLERGIES

Testing for allergies is done in two ways. The more sensitive method is to place a small quantity of the suspected allergen just under the skin with a syringe. If the individual is allergic to the material, a local reaction of redness, itching, and a small swelling will occur within 15 minutes.

A second way of testing for specific allergies is to test the patient's blood with RAST tests. These tests are not as sensitive as skin tests, but may be especially useful for young patients (under six years of age), who often cannot sit still for skin testing, or for patients who cannot be taken off antihistamines.

ALLERGY TREATMENTS

The best treatment is to avoid the suspected allergen. Because allergens such as grass, weeds, and house dust cannot be completely avoided, treatment with medications may be necessary. These medications are decongestants, antihistamines, and corticosteroids. Only the antihistamines would be containdicated in a person with Sjögren's syndrome. Antihistamines tend to cause dryness, the last thing a Sjögren's syndrome patient wants. Antihistamines may be used, if necessary and if given in a sufficiently low dosage.

Allergy shots help allergy sufferers, in part by reducing the quantity of IgE. This occurs over a period of several years, as the dosage of the allergy shots is increased. This form of therapy should be reserved for those patients who suffer from allergic symptoms that are not helped by medications or who have symptoms over a prolonged period of time, such as more than three weeks a year.

Patients may obtain symptomatic relief from allergic eye symptoms with Opticrom eye drops (Fisons Co.) These are not contraindicated in patients with SS.

Wide lens, wraparound goggles offer practical protection from allergens, such as pollen, mold, dander, and dust. These goggles can be obtained as sun goggles or as clear goggles that can be worn indoors. A mask may be worn as well on bad allergic days to reduce the exposure to allergens.

16

Pregnancy

Jill P. Buyon, M.D.

During the course of a normal pregnancy, antibodies in the mother's circulation are transported across the placenta into the bloodstream of the fetus. These antibodies protect the developing fetus, which is incapable of making its own antibodies against bacteria and viruses.

Unfortunately, in mothers with diseases such as systemic lupus erythematosus (SLE) and Sjögren's syndrome (SS), abnormal autoimmune antibodies directed against self-molecules can also cross the placenta and enter the fetal circulation. Certain of these autoantibodies are particularly detrimental to the fetus and can attack the developing heart tissue, resulting in permanent complete heart block, a potentially life-threatening condition.

In congenital complete heart block, the normal electrical signal stimulating and regulating the fetal heartbeat is in some way interrupted or damaged by the autoantibodies. Although the heart may still be stimulated at another excitation point, the baby's heartbeat will be abnormal.

The detrimental autoantibodies thus far identified by numerous investigators are those directed against normal cellular components called SS-A/Ro and SS-B/La. Curiously, these autoantibodies are associated with heart problems only in the child, not in the mother.

FETAL AND MATERNAL TESTING

The strong association between maternal autoantibodies to Ro and La and heart problems in the growing fetus calls attention to the necessity of fetal and maternal testing for mothers at risk of having affected children. Autoantibodies to Ro and La occur frequently in patients with confirmed Sjögren's syndrome. Therefore, it is prudent that all SS patients be tested prior to conception and monitored during pregnancy.

Because tests differ in their sensitivity, the method of testing is important. Some laboratories are capable of detecting even small amounts of these autoantibodies. This is important, because it is not currently clear whether it is solely the quantity of autoantibody or some as yet unknown quality of the autoantibody that is critical in causing fetal heart damage.

Right now, the most sensitive test involves an enzyme-linked immunosorbent assay (ELISA), in which the patient's serum is tested for autoantibodies against highly purified forms of Ro and La. This type of testing should be readily available at most university medical centers. The patient's serum can be safely sent by normal mail delivery to such centers as well.

WHAT ARE THE RISKS?

If a mother is found to have autoantibodies against Ro and La, what is her risk of giving birth to a child with a heart problem? Although the exact incidence is unknown and somewhat controversial, generally the chances are one in 60 pregnancies. This appears to be a low risk. However, it is higher than the reported incidence of heart block in the population at large, that is, in mothers without these autoantibodies.

As testing becomes more sophisticated, we may find that only mothers with autoantibodies to Ro or La or another antibody with a related specificity give birth to babies with heart block. This is an area of active investigation.

What should be done to prevent a problem, once the mother's risk is identified? This depends largely on whether this is a first pregnancy or whether the mother has already had a child born with heart block.

FIRST PREGNANCY

If this is a first pregnancy, a conservative approach is probably warranted. This should consist of serial ultrasonography of the developing fetus every few weeks after the tenth week of gestation, with very careful attention during the twentieth to twenty-fourth weeks.

Should a problem be detected in the fetal heart, therapies (described below) directed at lowering autoantibody levels or at simply attempting to treat the heart condition may be justified.[1]

Once established, however, heart block is not likely to be reversed, so this situation is a bit of a "Catch 22." At this point, the outcome ranges from in utero death to the birth of a child with heart block, who may require a lifetime pacemaker. In some fortunate cases, children can live normal lives without requiring a pacemaker.

Given the varying outcomes, the choice of management in a first pregnancy is a difficult one.

SUBSEQUENT PREGNANCIES

In a mother with known autoantibodies who has already had a child with heart block, the risk of having a second child with heart block may be as high as one in four. Does this justify ag-

---

[1]Buyon J, Swersky S, Fox H, Bierman F, Winchester, RJ: Intrauterine therapy for presumptive fetal myocarditis with acquired heart block due to systemic lupus erythamatosus: experience in a mother with a predominance of SS-B/La antibodies. *Arthritis Rheum* 1987, 30:44-49.

gressive management in the early weeks of pregnancy? This is extremely controversial.

Management involves the use of plasmapheresis and/or steroids. Plasmapheresis, a procedure in which the patient's blood is removed and "cleansed" of the autoantibody, is time-consuming, requiring up to three six-hour sessions per week. (There is no exchange of another person's blood.) While such an approach has been attempted successfully, experience with this procedure is still far too limited to be routinely recommended.

SUMMARY

Autoantibodies to Ro and La pose a risk, albeit small, to the developing fetus. Currently, numerous laboratories are investigating the mechanisms of this problem, in an attempt to more specifically identify high-risk pregnancies and to develop treatment plans that might prevent heart block in the fetus.

Part IV

Caring for Yourself

17

Living with a Chronic Disease

Mark Flapan, Ph.D.

This chapter has been adapted from an article published in a National Organization of Rare Disorders newsletter. Although written about the general experiences of persons living with a chronic disease, much of the article relates to persons with Sjögren's syndrome.

When family members or friends ask, "How are you?," they usually want to know if you are in any particular pain or discomfort or any better or worse physically than before. Seldom do they have in mind your emotional state. Yet emotional reactions to an illness are sometimes more stressful than the physical effects.

While you and your family are doing everything you can to treat and cope with the physical effects of a chronic disease, there is more you can do to relieve emotional distress. You can learn to better understand and accept your feelings, without shame, self-blame, guilt, or recrimination.

To promote this understanding, commonly experienced emotions of persons with a chronic illness will be described. While not

everyone experiences all of these reactions, many of these thoughts
and feelings have been felt, but never expressed or possibly even
acknowledged, by persons with a chronic disorder. Describing
these emotions may be upsetting to those of you who are able to
maintain a positive attitude by putting aside disturbing thoughts
and feelings.

By discussing the distressing emotions of anger, self-blame,
shame, frustration, self-devaluation, self-pity, guilt, and fear, this
chapter may provide the emotional relief of a shared understanding.

ANGER

You may be angry because you have a chronic illness. But at
whom should you be angry? God, fate, the whole world? You may
be angry at doctors, because they have no cure for your disorder.
You thought doctors knew so much, and now realize they don't.
What's more, your doctors may not seem particularly interested in
you, except as a "case." When you visit a physician, he or she may
be rushed and not explain enough to you or may say things that
upset and frighten you.

You may also be angry at family members and friends, who at
times are unavailable when you need them and who may expect
more of you than you are capable of doing. You may wish your
friends could live in your body for a day or even an hour, so they
could understand what life is like for those with an incurable
disorder. Then maybe they wouldn't say and do things that hurt
your feelings. You may also be upset by the thought that your
family and friends might resent all they have to do for you, and feel
hurt and resentful in return.

SELF-BLAME

You may blame yourself for your illness, suspecting that you
have brought on your symptoms by not taking proper care of
yourself. Or maybe God is punishing you for doing something

wrong, even though you don't know what. You just feel it's your own fault.

SHAME

If you take your illness as a sign of weakness or a reflection of a flawed character, you will be ashamed to be ill. If you pride yourself on being independent or on doing things for others, you may be especially ashamed when you need others to do things for you. Moreover, if you have a visible disfigurement or deformity, you may be painfully self-conscious and ashamed.

FRUSTRATION

If you have a disability that requires you to rely on others for your daily needs, you are constantly frustrated. You are frustrated because you cannot do these things for yourself and frustrated because others do not do them promptly enough or exactly as you would like. Also frustrating and depressing are the inability to engage in activities you once enjoyed and the loss of abilities in which you once took pride.

SELF-DEVALUATION

If you are unable to do what you used to do, you not only feel frustrated, but inadequate as well. If, in addition, you are a perfectionist with expectations that you can no longer meet, you may disparage and even hate yourself.

SELF-PITY

If you cannot lead a normal life like everyone else, you may feel sorry for yourself. You may feel cheated and unfairly treated, if are are unable to finish your education, get married, enjoy sexual relations, give birth to or take care of your children, earn a living, or pursue a career. It's difficult not to feel resentment and envy for others who can do all these things.

GUILT

You may feel guilty, if you cannot fulfill your responsibilities as a wife or husband. Guilt may be unbearable, if you are a mother unable to do all you think you should for your children. Guilt is intensified, if you feel you are a burden on others, especially if you need help in personal care and hygiene. Should you sense resentment on the part of family members on whom you depend, you will feel not only guilt, but hurt as well.

FEAR

When a chronic disorder is potentially progressive, you live in dread of the future and are alarmed by any actual or imagined change in the the course of your disease. Should your condition become life-threatening, a cloud hangs over your head. You are also plagued with fears related to your family. If you have young children, you worry about what will happen to them, should something happen to the you. If you are dependent on your parents or marital partner for personal care, you worry about what will happen to you, should anything happen to those who are caring for you. Although you know it is unlikely, you may wonder what would happen, if your partner were to get tired of taking care of you and leave. What would you do then?

EMOTIONAL RELIEF

Even though your emotional reactions may be commonplace, if you criticize yourself for your feelings, you will suffer more than need be. You can gain both understanding and self-acceptance by sharing your feelings with a sympathetic family member or friend who is sensitive to your feelings and who knows how to listen. You can even use this chapter as a basis for talking about your feelings.

Sjögren's syndrome patients can lighten their emotional burden by sharing their feelings in a "Moisture Seekers" support group or with others individually. If this is not sufficiently helpful, you can benefit from professional counselling. Counselling not only may relieve the pains of guilt, apprehension, anxiety, self-disparagement, and depression, but may provide new perspectives for living and coping with your illness.

No one is responsible for a chronic disease. But you are responsible for what you do and don't do to help yourself live with your disorder.

18

Nutrition

Eden Kalman, M.A., R.D.

Although diminished salivary gland secretion resulting in xerostomia (dry mouth) is only one of many distressing symptoms of Sjögren's syndrome (SS), this particular symptom is the focal point when addressing the nutritional needs and concerns often associated with SS. Salivary insufficiency can result in difficulty in chewing and swallowing; adherence of food to the buccal (cheek) surfaces; fissures and ulcers of the tongue, mucous membranes, and lips, particularly at the corners of the mouth; rampant dental decay; and altered taste sensation.

These problems can markedly affect an adequate intake of nutritious foods. When the diet is inadequate to meet bodily requirements, the individual is not as healthy as he or she could be. This, in turn, may affect nutritional status and therefore one's ability to cope with the physical and emotional stress of Sjögren's syndrome.

Here are some considerations for a nutritious, well-balanced diet and suggestions, recommendations, and information that may assist in solving specific problems related to (1) chewing and swallowing difficulties caused by dryness and soreness, (2) dental-health, and (3) altered taste sensations.

A NUTRITIOUS, WELL-BALANCED DIET

A nutritious, well-balanced diet consists of a variety of foods in combination with a recommended number of servings from the four basic food groups: meat, milk, fruits and vegetables, and grains.

(1) The *meat group* consists not only of beef, lamb, and pork, but also of poultry, fish, eggs, and protein equivalents, such as nuts and dried legumes. Two, two-ounce servings every day provide good sources of protein, niacin, iron, and thiamine (vitamin B1).

(2) *Milk, hard cheese, yogurt,* and *calcium equivalents,* such as cottage cheese, provide calcium, phosphorous, and riboflavin, as well as protein. A *minimum* of two cups of milk or yogurt or two ounces of cheese are recommended daily for most adults. Four or more servings are recommended for women who are predisposed to osteoporosis (thinning of the bones) or who have been diagnosed as having this disorder.

Some individuals must avoid milk and milk products, because they have a lactose intolerance, that is, an intolerance to milk sugar and therefore to milk and milk products. This intolerance is caused by a deficiency of the enzyme lactase, which is essential for absorption of lactose from the gastrointestinal tract. Lactose intolerance is characterized by gastrointestinal symptoms, such as diarrhea and flatulence (excessive gas in the stomach and intestines).

When milk and milk products are eliminated from the diet, excellent sources of calcium are eliminated, also. Once a lactose intolerance is diagnosed by a physician (M.D.), a registered dietitian (R.D.) should be consulted to plan a nutritious diet that meets individual needs. Depending on the level of intolerance, alternatives to milk include:
• trying smaller portions of milk and milk products
• consuming milk and milk products in combination with other foods (e.g., macaroni and cheese casserole)
• hard cheeses, which contain smaller amounts of lactose
• lactose reduced milk
• lactose reduced cheese

- for a more severe lactose intolerance, lact-aid enzyme can be taken orally or added to milk to reduce the lactose content of milk or to aid in the digestion of lactose
- a calcium supplement, such as Oscal or Tums (calcium carbonate), may be indicated, when the alternatives above do not provide relief from the symptoms of lactose intolerance

(3) *Fruits and vegetables* contain carbohydrate, fiber, iron, and vitamins A and C. Four or more servings are recommended daily. This should include at least one source of vitamin C (grapefruit, orange, cantaloupe, strawberries, brocolli, or green peppers). A good source of vitamin A (dark green or yellow vegetables) should be eaten several times a week.

(4) Besides bread and cereal, the *breads and cereals group* includes pasta and rice. Eating more whole grain breads, cereals, and grain products increases dietary fiber and tends to reduce problems such as chronic constipation. In addition to fiber, many essential B vitamins, some protein, iron, and minerals are also provided. Four or more servings are recommended daily.

In addition to the four food groups, another food category includes sugar, sugar products, oils, fats, and alcoholic beverages. Although they are tasty, these foods provide little other than calories from carbohydrates and fats. They should be eliminated from the diet, if ideal weight is desired or dental health is of concern. Otherwise, moderate consumption is recommended.

Although it is possible to get all nutrients required by eating a variety of foods from each of the four food groups every day, many individuals still choose to supplement their diet with vitamins for a variety of reasons. Should a supplement be desired or recommended, select a balanced multivitamin that provides approximately 100% of the recommended dietary allowance (RDA) of recognized nutrients established by the Nutrition Board of the National Academy of Sciences.

Large doses or megadoses (10 times the RDA) are unnecessary, unless prescribed by a physician. Otherwise, they are potentially harmful and should be avoided. Because fat-soluble vitamins (A,D, E, and K) are stored in the body, excessive intake may lead to toxic buildup. Water-soluble vitamins, once thought to be safe, because they are usually excreted by the kidneys, may also cause trouble, if excessive amounts are ingested for prolonged periods of time.

The following information is reprinted with permission from the *Gastroenterology Newsletter,* published by Seymour Katz, M.D. and Arthur L. Talansky, M.D.:

"*Vitamin A* (RDA = 1,000 I.U./day): The average American diet contains 5,000 to 10,000 units/day. When greater than 25,000 to 50,000 I.U. are taken for months, changes occur in the form of dry, scaling skin, hair loss, itching, soreness of tongue and mouth, brittle nails, altered eye muscle movements, dangerous levels of calcium in blood, increased size and scar tissue of liver and spleen, increased pressure in the brain, and fever. Children may become irritable with tender bones and fail to gain weight.

"*Vitamin D* (RDA = 400 I.U.): This is the most common of the vitamins involved in overdosage. If exceeding 60,000 I.U. daily, the result may be muscle weakness, headache, nausea, vomiting, bone pain, high levels of blood calcium and calcium deposits, increased urinary protein, high blood pressure, and cardiac rhythm disturbances. Ultimately, calcium deposits progress in blood vessels and may lead to kidney failure.

"*Vitamin E* (RDA = 15 I.U.): Although large doses are usually well tolerated, muscle weakness, fatigue, and nausea may occur with doses as low as 300 to 800 I.U./day. Larger doses have led to cramps, diarrhea, and interference with the blood clotting system. This is particularly important for patients taking anticoagulant therapy.

"*Vitamin K:* Large doses in pregnancy have led to jaundiced newborns and interference with anticoagulant therapy in some patients. (Lee M, *Ann Intern Med* 94:140, 1981.)

"Recent work with water-soluble vitamins has raised serious concern with vitamins heretofore considered 'safe.'

"*Vitamin B6* (Pyridoxine) (RDA = 2.2 mg./day): Twenty mg. has been taken without ill effect, but severe nerve disorders have developed in patients taking B6 in 'gram' quantities. These problems included numbness, awkward movements of limbs, loss of vibration sense, impaired perceptions of touch and temperature, with lost reflexes. Fortunately, all are reversible with discontinuing the medication. (Shaumberg H, *New Engl J Med* 310:198, 1984.) This vitamin in low doses (25 mg./day) can interfere with Levodopa therapy and thereby decrease its effectiveness in Parkinson's disease, as well as reduce the anticonvulsant effect of Dilantin or barbiturates.

"*Vitamin C* (RDA = 60 mg./day): Long considered sacred in large doses, it may produce diarrhea with as little as 1 gm. per day, increase uric acid in urine with 4 gms. daily, and may lead to urinary oxalate stones or break down red blood cells in certain patients with inherited blood disorders, for example, G6PD deficiency. Large doses may interfere with oral anticoagulation treatment and enhance toxic effects of estrogens.

"*Nicotinic acid* (Niacin) (RDA = 13 to 19 mg./day): Larger doses have been used to lower serum cholesterol or treat certain psychiatric diseases. The flushing, itching, and intestinal complaints are due to Niacin releasing histamine from the body. This may aggravate existing asthma, increase uric acid leading to gout, and elevate blood sugars. (*JAMA* 231:360, 1975.) Liver toxicity with jaundice may occur with as little as 750 mg. daily."

SUGGESTIONS FOR SOLVING CHEWING AND SWALLOWING PROBLEMS CAUSED BY SORENESS AND DRYNESS

(1) Modify your diet to include foods of a softer consistency. Continue making the foods you like, but use a blender, food processor, or Crock-Pot, with extra liquids, gravies, sauces, or broth to soften or liquify foods.

(2) Consider foods you like that are naturally soft, such as cooked eggs, cheeses (if tolerated), simmered stews, casseroles, and pasta dishes. Milk products, such as yogurt, instant breakfast, milkshake, pudding, custard, and ice cream, if tolerated, are soft and nutritious. Include mashed potato, rice, cooked creamy cereals, banana, canned fruit, and fruit nectars.

(3) Avoid spices, such as pepper, chili powder, nutmeg, and cloves, and acidic fruit juices. These may irritate buccal surfaces.

(4) Avoid dry foods, such as breads and crackers, or soak them in your favorite liquid.

(5) Eat foods at a comfortable temperature, usually cool or warm, rather than cold or hot.

(6) Drink plenty of fluids with meals. This eases chewing and swallowing and increases the taste of food.

(7) If needed, medical nutritional supplements (e.g., Sustacal, Ensure) can be prescribed to provide adequate intake of calories and nutrients.

SUGGESTIONS FOR MAINTAINING DENTAL HEALTH

(1) Eat a variety of foods and the recommended number of servings from the basic four food groups: meat, milk, fruits and vegetables, and grains to provide nutrients essential to preventing gum disease and tooth decay.

(2) Avoid simple carbohydrates, such as sucrose (table sugar), fructose, sugary foods, and highly processed refined foods made from starches, which often contain significant amounts of sugars.

(3) Avoid sweets, especially when snacking between meals. Instead, include foods with protein and/or fat (e.g., cheese), which neutralize acid and help protect teeth.

(4) Avoid sweet/sticky foods, such as chewy candy, hard candy, dried fruits, cookies, and syrupy toppings. Substitute these sweets with *sugarless* gums and candies. Chewing and sucking help to stimulate saliva.

(5) If tolerated, eat raw fruits and vegetables. Foods high in fiber content help stimulate salivation, a factor in preventing tooth decay.

SUGGESTIONS FOR COPING WITH
ALTERED TASTE SENSATION

(1) Avoid foods that you find offensive.

(2) Experiment with new seasonings and new food combina-

tions. Try new recipes with ingredients that you tolerate well.

(3) Experiment with food temperature.

(4) An increased consumption of liquids (unsweetened only) at or between meals may remove offensive mouth tastes.

(5) Chew sugarless gums and suck sugarless candy. These leave their own taste.

(6) Rule out dental problems that may cause a bad taste. See your dentist on a routine basis.

SUGGESTIONS FOR FURTHER READING

Smith SM, A new approach to vitamin supplementation. *Environmental Nutrition Newsletter,* Vol. 7, No. 4, 1984, p. 1-2.

Burakoff RP, Nutritional guidelines for oral health. *Environmental Nutrition Newsletter,* Vol. 7, No. 11, 1984, p. 1-2.

A subscription to *Environmental Nutrition Newsletter* is available by writing: Environmental Nutrition, 2112 Broadway, Suite 200, New York, NY 10023. Phone: (212) 362-0424.

Arthritis Diet and Nutrition—Facts to Consider. Arthritis Foundation. This publication is available from the Arthritis Foundation, 3400 Peachtree Road, N.E., Atlanta, GA 30326.

Skinner S and Martens RA, *The Milk Sugar Dilemma: Living with Lactose Intolerance.* Medi-Ed Press, 1985. Medi-Ed Press, P.O. Box 957, East Lansing, MI 48823.

Eating Hints—Recipes and Tips for Better Nutrition During Treatment. U. S. Department of Health, Education, and Welfare. NIH Publication No. 80-2079, January, 1980. For copies, write: Office of Cancer Communications, National Cancer Institute, Bethesda, MD 20205.

A Guide to Good Eating—A Recommended Daily Pattern. National Dairy Council, 1984.

Nutrition and Your Health—Dietary Guidelines for Americans. U. S. Department of Agriculture and U. S. Department of Health and Human Services, February, 1980.

Rodnam GP and Schumacher HR, eds. *Primer on the Rheumatic Diseases,* 8th edition. Arthritis Founation, 1983. (Catalog No. 3250.)

19

Voice

Joan Levy, M.A., C.C.C. in Speech

Voice is an integral part of our lives. Yet we do not fully appreciate it until a problem arises and we cannot speak comfortably or at all.

The lack of saliva in Sjögren's syndrome (SS) patients and resulting dry mouth may cause voice problems. Dry vocal cords do not always come together properly; this leads to vocal fatigue and voice fade-out. When the SS patient then tries to "push out" the voice by changing pitch or by force, the voice becomes hoarse. The person with SS may clear his or her throat frequently, causing excessive pressure on the vocal cords. Redness and edema (excessive fluid accumulation) may occur.

HOW IS VOICE PRODUCED NORMALLY?

The vocal cords act as a sound source to produce voice. In inhalation, air goes through the nose and mouth into the larynx; the vocal cords move apart and air travels down the respiratory mechanism until it reaches the lungs. Exhalation movement brings the vocal cords together. Any alterations of mass, elasticity, or compliance can cause a vocal problem.

WHAT ARE VOICE DISORDERS?

A voice disorder can be broadly defined as something that interferes with smooth, effortless sound. Voice problems are divided into the following categories:

(1) Pitch: too high, too low, falsetto, diplophonia (production of double sounds).

(2) Intensity: too loud, too soft.

(3) Resonance: nasal, denasal.

(4) Quality: harsh (voice sounds raspy and can result in "vocal fry" or very low-pitched, tired, weak voice); breathy (bowed vocal cords do not close and air escapes); and hoarse (a combination of harsh and breathy). Fatigue increases vocal fry.

Subjective descriptions such as "harsh," "hoarse," and "breathy," are instantaneous reactions to what is heard. In recent years, voice laboratories have provided more objective measurements of voice quality.

ORGANIC AND FUNCTIONAL VOICE DISORDERS

Although voice disorders fall into two classifications, organic (physical causes) and functional (emotional and/or behavioral causes), the two are interactive. For example, abuse of the voice can lead to growths, which then make the problem physical. Or an organic cause can be cured, but a residual voice problem may remain.

TYPES OF ORGANIC VOICE PROBLEMS

(1) Tumors are cancerous or benign growths. Nodules, polyps, and contact ulcers are always benign.

(2) Papillomas are viral: warts, herpes.

(3) Paralyzed vocal cord: from surgery, viral infection, or injury. Recovery is sometimes spontaneous.

(4) Systemic: results from a generalized disease, such as Sjögren's syndrome, which attacks different parts of the body. A dry larynx may become swollen and fatigued, so that when the patient coughs or clears the throat, the vocal cords are irritated.

(5) Neurological causes.

(6) Respiratory disorders.

VOICE THERAPY

Voice therapy helps maximize the voice by teaching strategies for more effective voice production. A trained listener is advantageous, providing control and helping the patient monitor his or her own speech. Direct voice therapy should not continue indefinitely, but only as long as needed to achieve the two goals of treatment: counselling and direct work on symptoms.

Counselling: The voice therapist discusses the where, why, and how of individual voice abuse and misuse with the patient, helping him or her to eliminate or reduce adverse situations, such as clearing the throat and trying to talk too much at one time. Other forms of vocal abuse include smoking; consumption of excessive alcohol and caffeine; and certain medications, such as decongestants and diuretics, which may cause or exacerbate dryness. Situations where misuse of the voice may be more subtle, such as excessive use of the telephone and visiting noisy restaurants, should be avoided, also.

Direct strategies for working on the voice include:

(1) Using aids such as a microphone and tape recorder.

(2) Developing more effective breathing patterns for speech by working on phrasing and pausing.

(3) Using relaxation techniques to reduce head, neck, and bodily tension.

(4) Eliminating the hard glottal attack when starting to speak, and using instead one of the "yawn-sigh" aspiration words that begin with an "h," such as "how," "happy," or "who." Do not start speaking with words beginning with a hard consonant, such as "give" or "come." Although open mouth breathing is contraindicated in patients with SS, because of the difficulty they have with the open mouth drying up so quickly, modifications of the "yawn-sigh" exercises are needed. If patients push words out, their vocal cords will become irritated, exacerbating the problem.

(5) Work on phrasing and pausing, which teaches one not to talk on residual air. When one tries to push on to say more, without stopping for air, the cords suffer more strain and abuse. This may result in vocal fade-out.

(6) Work on production with various vowel sounds, some of which are anti-harsh. This helps with easy onset of speech, which in turn reduces abuse to the vocal cords.

HELPFUL SUGGESTIONS

(1) Sipping water provides temporary relief for voice problems caused by dryness.

(2) Using a humidifier at home helps keep air moist.

(3) Nasal breathing is better than open mouth breathing. In relaxation exercises, breathe in and out through the nose.

(4) Since salivary glands in Sjögren's syndrome patients produce only a limited amount of saliva, the stimulation provided by sugarless chewing gum may improve what production there is.

(5) Avoid clearing the throat by sipping water, sucking on a hard, sugarless candy, or simply swallowing. If clearing the throat cannot be prevented, using an "h" sound sound or humming will soften the attack on the vocal cords.

(6) When patients have trouble getting a word out, they may fear losing their voice altogether. Although losing the voice completely is rare, the emotional element of fear affects voice production. When having trouble getting a word out, try an easy onset "h" word, a humming sound, or laugh.

(6) Use a nasal douche before going to bed. Keep a humidifier on while sleeping; open mouth breathing during sleep dries out the throat and larynx.

(6) In speaking to a group, as opposed to social conversation with one or two friends, speak for a limited time and use a microphone. Speak in a small room, where the audience will be close.

(7) Keep a vocal log, charting daily voice use in various situations.

20

Nasal Irrigation

The following chapter has been adapted from a National Institutes of Health (NIH) Clinical Center publication, "Facts About the Nose and Nasal Irrigation," developed by Peggy Coleman, B.S.N., and Nancy Stefan, B.S.N.

The nose is composed of bone and cartilage, covered by skin on the outside and lined with mucous membrane. The nasal cavities are separated by a partition called the septum, which is usually bent more to one side so that the nasal cavities are not of equal size. This is important to remember when irrigating the nose, because each side will not irrigate the same way.

The roof of the nasal cavity has a slope that corresponds to the slope of the nasal bridge. Further back on the roof are the olfactory nerves. These are connected to the brain. On the ends of these nerves are the olfactory filaments that pick up odors. Not all air going through the nasal cavity reaches this area. Sniffing will create currents that carry odor upward to the olfactory mucosa. When air is exhaled, it does not pass this area. This is why one cannot smell anything when exhaling.

Each chamber of the nose is divided into many spaces by bony ridges called turbinates, which extend down from the sides of the nose. These turbinates have openings that drain the sinuses. The mucous membrane in the nose also lines the sinuses. Cilia (very fine microscopic hairs) in the mucous membrane move back and forth, creating a movement of mucus from the sinuses into the nasal cavity. The tear ducts also empty into the nasal cavity.

The mucous lining of the nose has many tiny blood vessels close to the surface. This is why the nose bleeds so easily when injured or when the mucous membrane becomes dry. The mucous membranes secrete about a quart of fluid daily, much of it humidifying the air entering the throat and lungs. Individuals with chronic nasal and sinus disease frequently require additional room humidification.

Patients with Sjögren's syndrome often have problems with drying of the nasal mucosa. Because the secretion of mucus is thick, and the cilia do not effectively move it, the mucus dries and forms crusts. These crusts can interfere with sinus drainage, often leading to sinus pain, headaches, infection, and bad odors.

Patients have found that instilling nose drops to lubricate and moisten the mucosa helps to diminish the incidence of crusting. Some patients have to irrigate the nasal mucosa to remove crusts. Patients who do irrigate with warm, normal saline say that irrigating relieves their congestion, as well as the discomfort caused by congestion.

INSTRUCTIONS FOR NASAL IRRIGATION

Purposes:

(1) To remove crusts, mucus, and secretions from the nasal passages, thereby reducing risk of infection and increasing comfort and breathing ease.

(2) To relieve inflammation and congestion of the nasal mucosa.

Equipment needed:

(1) Small bulb syringe or electric dental device.

(2) Irrigation tips—rigid or flexible, depending on preference.

(3) Warm saline solution and a thermometer. Make the saline solution according to the instructions at the end of this chapter. Heat the water in a pan. Have a thermometer handy to measure the temperature, which should be 103°-105° F. or 39.4°-41.6° C. Either tap or distilled water can be used.

(4) Plastic sheet, apron, or towel to protect clothing.

(5) Box of facial tissues for disposal of loosened mucus, crusts, or secretions.

(6) Acetic acid solution (0.25%) to rinse bulb syringe or dental device after irrigation. See instructions at the end of this chapter.

(7) Basin or sink for collection of used irrigating solution and materials and fluid expelled from the nose during irrigation.

Step-by-step instructions:

(1) Wash hands.

(2) Find a comfortable place to sit, so that the irrigating tip can reach into the nose and the irrigation return can flow into the basin or sink. If using an electric dental device, sit conveniently near an power outlet.

(3) Sitting upright, bend the head forward over the basin and keep head well flexed on the chest. The nose and ear should be kept on a vertical plane. This will prevent inhaling the solution and will keep the Eustachian tube (between the ear and throat) above the level of the stream of solution.

(4) Before beginning the irrigation, rinse the syringe or electric dental device by running approximately one cup of normal saline though it. This will remove any residual acetic acid solution or debris and warm the tubing.

(5) Adjust the irrigation instrument on the lowest possible setting, and gradually increase the pressure only enough to achieve a steady, gentle, pulsating stream of warm water. The greater the force of the solution, the greater the possibility of driving material from the nose into the sinuses or Eustachian tube.

(6) Before irrigating, remember the following DO's and DON'Ts:

(a) DO keep your mouth open and breathe rhythmically though the mouth. This allows the soft palate to close off the throat and the stream of irrigating solution to flow back out the opposite nostril, bringing the discharge with it.

(b) DO remove the irrigating tip from the nostril, if you have to sneeze or cough. Removal of the irrigating tip will prevent accidental injury to the nasal mucosa.

(c) DON'T speak or swallow during the irrigation. Changes of pressure within the oral or nasal cavity could result in infectious material being drawn into the sinuses or Eustachian tube.

(7) Insert the nasal irrigation tip into the nostril, approximately one-half to one inch. The tip should be inserted far enough to promote cleansing of the mucosa. Squeeze the bulb syringe or turn on the electric irrigating device. Begin irrigating. Use 500 to 1,000 cc. of normal saline. The amount of fluid needed will vary, depending on the amount of crusting. Irrigate both nostrils.

(8) Wait a few minutes before blowing excess fluid from both nostrils simultaneously. Fluid will drain from the nose during that few minutes. Blowing through both nostrils prevents fluid and pressure from building up in the sinuses and Eustachian tubes. Gentle blowing helps loosen and expel crusts and mucus.

(9) Run approximately one cup of acetic acid solution (0.25%) through the machine and tubing, including the irrigating tip. Shake excess moisture from the parts and dry thoroughly. This prevents organisms from growing in the tubing.

Important: Observe the return solution for any change. Changes in the return of the cleansing solution can signal infection and should be reported to one's physician.

DIRECTIONS FOR MAKING SALINE
IRRIGATING SOLUTION (one liter)

Equipment needed:
(1) A one-liter plastic bottle or any clean container will a well-fitted cap.

(2) Common table salt, uniodized.

(3) A plastic medicine cup for measuring. A household teaspoon can be used, but may be less accurate.

To make the solution:

(1) Rinse out the plastic bottle with water. Any clean container with a well-fitted cap will do.

(2) Fill medicine cup to the 1/4-fluid-ounce mark with salt or use 1 1/2 teaspooonful.

(3) Pour salt into liter plastic bottle.

(4) Fill bottle with tap water up to the one-liter marking. Four cups and one ounce of water is approximately equal to 1,000 cc. Because the chlorine in tap water can be irritating to mucosa, some patients prefer distilled water.

(5) Shake until salt is dissolved.

DIRECTIONS FOR MAKING ACETIC ACID SOLUTION (0.25%)

Equipment needed:

(1) A one-liter plastic bottle or any clean container with a well-fitted plastic cap.

(2) Plain white vinegar.

(3) A small measuring cup or bottle.

To make the solution:

(1) Rinse the liter plastic bottle with water.

(2) Measure 50 milliliters (or 1 1/2 ounces) of vinegar and pour into bottle.

(3) Fill plastic liter bottle with water up to the liter mark. Four cups plus one ounce of water is approximately equal to 1,000 cc.

(4) Put the top on the liter bottle and shake.

21

Tips for More Comfortable Living

Elaine K. Harris

Most of the information in this chapter is based on material that has appeared in various issues of *The Moisture Seekers Newsletter*. Ruth Thompson, a member of the Pittsburgh Chapter of the Sjogren's Syndrome Foundation, was very helpful in assisting in the gathering of this material.

The information on taking medications and on stopping nose-bleeds originally appeared in issues of the University of California at Berkeley *Wellness Letter*. It appeared in *The Moisture Seekers Newsletter* with permission of the publisher.

TIPS FOR A MORE COMFORTABLE MOUTH
(See also Chapter 5)

To sooth dry lips, tongue, mouth:
- Apply thin coat of Vaseline, Crisco, or vegetable oil on lip area only.
- Apply Borofax (a lanolin-based emollient) or Oralbalance.
- Spread vitamin E inside mouth, especially before retiring for night. Use liquid or break capsule in the mouth; discard capsule. Provides a protective, soothing coating, which is unlikely to evaporate. Can be used during the day, also.

- Drink water; suck on ice cubes.
- To break up thick, mucouslike saliva in the mouth, use either saline solution (1/4 teaspoon salt to one cup of water) or Alkalol.

To preserve and protect tooth enamel:
- Use .4% stannous fluoride gel. Important that fluoride be neutral, not acidic. Gel-Kam (Sherer Laboratories); need prescription.
- Use remineralizing solutions, such as Salminsol Home Treatment Program. Order from:

> Dental Prophylaxis Systems, Inc.
> P. O. Box 3183
> Iowa City, IA 52244

Also available through *SMART MOUTH* catalog. This free catalog lists many dry mouth products, such as artificial salivas, dry mouth toothpaste, and special enzyme replacement chewing gum. Order from:

> SMART MOUTH
> Nuperco, Inc.
> P. O. Box 689
> 799 Franklin Ave.
> Franklin Lakes, NJ 07417
> Phone: (201) 891-7027

- Use dental floss between teeth at least once daily.
- Use toothpaste containing fluoride and consult with your dentist concerning the use of topical fluoride.
- See your dentist at least three times a year for a cleaning and early treatment of cavities.
- Try to avoid sticky, sugary foods.
- Brush teeth immediately after eating.

To relieve dryness:
- Take frequent sips of water or *sugarless* carbonated drinks. Many patients find diet soft drinks provide a better feeling of wetness than water.
- Pause often while speaking to sip some liquid.
- Chew gum, sugarless only (Biotene, Trident, and others). In Ca-

nada, Trident gum is available with xylitol, which is considered beneficial. Chewing may help produce more saliva. (See report on gum chewing in *The Moisture Seekers Newsletter,* May, 1988.)
- Suck on a small piece of lemon rind, fruit pit, mints, or sugarless hard candies—mint or lemon flavors are generally more effective. The sucking action helps stimulate saliva. Xylitol mints (available in Canada) and gum are also helpful in caries prevention.
- Keep a glass or carafe of water by your bed for dryness during the night or on awakening.
- Drink frequently while eating. This will make chewing and swallowing easier and may increase the taste of foods.
- Avoid coffee, tea, and other caffeinated drinks. Many patients report increased dryness after drinking caffeinated beverages.
- Investigate use of Salitron, an electronic device that stimulates the salivary glands. Information available from:

> Biosonics, Inc.
> 14000 D Commerce Parkway
> Mt. Laurel, NJ 08054
> Phone: (800) 547-4357

To relieve pain in parotid salivary gland area:
- Try gently massaging the area just below the bottom of the ear lobe with the fleshy part of your index and middle fingers, going forward to the end of the jawbone, slightly downward and over the jawbone, and up again towards the tip of the ear lobe. This sometimes helps to break loose a plug of mucus in the duct, thus relieving the pain caused by the blockage.

To combat Candida buildup in mouth:
- Gyne-Lotrimin or Nystatin vaginal tablets, which are available by prescription only, used orally are much more effective than liquid suspension or troches. Dissolve these vaginal tablets slowly in the mouth over 15 to 30 minutes.
- Peridex prescription medication.
- Not recommended: (1) Mycelex oral troches, which contain too

much glucose; (2) Nystatin oral suspension, which is a sucrose solution.

For angular cheilitis:
• Lotrimin or Mycelog ointment, both prescription medications. Inside of mouth must be treated simultaneously. (See tips for treating Candida.)

Special toothpastes:
• Biotene, Viadent, and Arm & Hammer.

Mouthwash:
• Dissolve 1/4 to 1/2 teaspoon of baking soda in 1/4 to 1/2 cup of warm water. This changes the pH balance and sweetens the mouth after eating foods that cause a bad aftertaste.
• Frequent rinsing with a solution of 1/2 teaspoon salt dissolved in glass of warm water will help break up thick mucus in mouth, which occurs because mucous-producing cells tend to be affected to a lesser degree than serous (water-producing) cells.

TIPS FOR A MORE COMFORTABLE NOSE
(See also Chapter 6)

To relieve dryness:
• Keep nasal passages moist by frequent use of nasal saline solution. These are available over-the-counter (OTC). Some of the brands are: Ayr, NaSal, Ocean, and Salinex.
• For severe head and nasal dryness, irrigate the nose daily:
    (1) with nasal douche (glass or plastic); use either a solution of Alkalol with water (two parts Alkalol to one part water) or saline solution (1/4 teaspoon salt to one cup water).
    (2) use a Water Pik with nasal irrigator attachment and saline solution (1/4 teaspooon salt to one cup water) to clean out dried mucus in upper nasal passage. Attachment can be ordered from:
            Ethicare
            P. O. Box 5027
            Fort Lauderdale, FL 33310
            Phone: (305) 742-3599

(See also Chapter 20, Nasal Irrigation.)
- Apply vitamine E oil or Borofax to rim of nostrils only. *Do not put up nose.*
- Use a cool vapor humidifier to prevent dry air during indoor heating season. Clean regularly to prevent mold and mildew. Distilled water should be used for filling ultrasonic humidifiers, or obtain one that has a demineralization cartridge. Also check with your doctor about use of ultrasonic humidifiers. (See September, 1988, *Consumer Reports* article on humidifiers.)
- Avoid petroleum-based products, such as Vaseline, other than at the tip of nostrils, since use in nasal passages can result in aspiration into lungs.
- Use Borofax at rim of nostrils at bedtime and when necessary during the day.
- Use a car humidifier. The Miniature Sunbeam ultrasonic humidifier is used with inverter that plugs into car cigarette lighter. (Power Verter Model PV 100, DC to AC, 100 watts, manufactured by: Trippe Lite, Division of Trippe Manufacturing Co., Chicago, IL 60610. Cost: About $70 at time of publication.)
- If nose is too dry to blow, use a moistened cotton swab just inside the nostrils to help remove dried up mucus.

To stop a nosebleed quickly:
- Sit up so that gravity will lower pressure in the veins. To keep blood from running back into the throat, tilt the head forward a little.
- Pinch the fleshy part of the nose between the bridge and nostrils with the thumb and index finger for five to 10 minutes. Applying ice probably won't help, since it is really pressure that does the trick.
- If pressure alone does not work, wet a cotton or tissue plug with Afrin, Neosynephrine, or similar decongestant nasal solution, insert into the nose about one inch, and then reapply pressure.
- After bleeding stops, don't blow the nose too hard or too often. Sneeze through an open mouth, and avoid strenuous sports for a few days. Apply a little lubricant (Borofax, Vaseline, or similar lubricant) just inside the nostrils with a small cotton swab,

several times a day for a week, to keep membranes moist. If nose bleeds on plane trips, use this technique before departure. (See tips on plane travel.)

TIPS FOR MORE COMFORTABLE EYES
(See also Chapter 4)

- Soaking Lacriserts for 10 or 15 minutes in nonpreserved artifical tears may make them more comfortable to use.
- Containers for keeping nonpreserved eye drops:
  (1) Thermos model #3700, 10 oz. "Roughneck Flip & Sip." Contains no glass. Tall enough to hold bottle of Dessel's Gum Cellulose Tears plus two ice cubes; $5. *Dessel's Pharmacy* compounds and ships many hard-to-obtain prescription medications, including Mucomyst and nonpreserved gum cellulose in .3, .625, .95, and 1.25%, and stocks many other over-the-counter items helpful to SS patients. For information:

  > Dessel's Pharmacy
  > 756 Irving St.
  > San Francisco, CA 94112
  > Phone: (415) 681-3300

  (2) Aladdin 6 oz., foam-insulated thermos jar with freezer lid (lid can be placed in freezer, and then serves as a coolant).
  (3) Medicool. Available from:

  > Eagle Vision
  > 6485 Poplar Ave.
  > Memphis, TN 38119
  > Phone: (800) 222-PLUG

- Keeping your eyes closed for three minutes, if possible, after inserting eye drops increases their effectiveness and decreases their absorption systemically.
- Wraparound sun goggles called "SuperVisors" have side shields and can be worn over prescription glasses. They are not recom-

mended for use at night and are not to be worn as safety glasses. 1988 cost: $18.50 + $2.50 shipping. Other companies make similar goggles.

"SuperVisors" can be ordered from:

> Eye Communications
> 1209 South Shamrock
> Monrovia, CA 91016
> Phone: (818) 358-1841

In the treatment of blepharitis:
• To keep compresses hot for the recommended 10- to 20-minute treatment, use a first aid gel pack that has been heated and then wrapped in two thick, heavy, clean washcloths. Lie down, apply the pack to your eyes, and relax. Listen to music.
• To clean eyelids and lashes, wipe with a mixture of equal parts of warm water and baby shampoo. This may cause irritation to susceptible individuals.
• Some commercial preparations for cleaning your eyelids: I-Scrub, manufactured by Spectra, (800)-225-2578; OCuSoft Lid Scrub, manufactured by OCuSoft, Inc., (800) 233-5469. These products may not yet be available in your local pharmacy.

General recommendations for the proper use of eye drops and ointments (courtesy of Dessel's Pharmacy):

Eye drops:
• Wash hands thoroughly.
• Gently pull lower eyelid down.
• Lie down or tilt head backward and look at ceiling; hold dropper above eye, drop medicine inside lower lid while looking up.
• Do not touch dropper to eye, fingers, or any surface.
• Release lower lid. Try to keep eye open and not blink for at least 30 seconds.
• Apply gentle pressure with fingers to bridge of nose (inside corner of the eye) for about one minute to prevent drainage of solution from intended area.
• If dropper is separate, hold it with tip down. Replace on bottle and tighten cap.

- Never rinse dropper.
- Never use eye drops that have changed color.
- If you are using more than one kind of drop at the same time, wait at least five minutes before using other drops.

Eye ointments (emollients):
- Wash hands thoroughly.
- To improve flow of ointment, hold tube in hand several minutes to warm before use.
- Gently pull lower eyelid down.
- Lie back or tilt head backward and look at ceiling; squeeze a small amount of ointment (about 1/4 to 1/2 inch) inside lower lid.
- Close eye gently and roll eyeball in all directions while eye is closed. Temporary blurring may occur.
- When opening ointment tube for the first time, squeeze out the first 1/4 inch of ointment and discard, as it may be too dry.
- If you are using more than one kind of ointment at the same time, wait about 10 minutes before using other ointment.

TIPS FOR A MORE COMFORTABLE VAGINA
(See also Chapter 8)

- Use only water-soluble lubricants in the vagina, such as K-Y Jelly; H-R Jelly; Surgilube (more viscous), manufactured by E. Fougera & Co., Melville, NY 11747; Maxilube (the most viscous), manufactured by Mission Pharmacal Co., San Antonio, TX 78296.
- Apply vitamin E oil, which is helpful in keeping vaginal tissue soft. Break open a vitamin E capsule and squeeze contents on labia. Vitamin E oil and creams are also available, but may contain preservatives that can prove irritating. Vitamin E suppositories are available from some health food stores, but usually not found in pharmacies; contain preservatives that can prove irritating.

TIPS FOR MORE COMFORTABLE SKIN
(See also Chapter 9)

Most of the following information is excerpted from the June, 1988, *Moisture Seekers Newsletter* report on a presentation by Pamela B. Tripp, M.D.

- Avoid harsh antibacterial soaps, such as Coast, Dial, Irish Spring, Ivory, Lifebuoy, Safeguard, Shield, and Zest. Use soaps such as Alpha Keri, Basis, Caress, Dove, Lowila, Neutragena Dry Skin Soap, Oilatum, and Purpose, or use soap substitutes such as Aquinil, Cetaphil, or SFC lotions.
- Avoid excessive bathing (more than one bath a day). If you take a bath daily, soak in a tub of warm water for 10 to 15 minutes to hydrate the skin. When you get out of the shower or bath, do not dry off completely; leave a film of moisture and then apply the cheapest lubricant you can find.
- Bath oils recommended by Dr. Tripp include Alpha Keri, Aveeno, Domol, Herbal, and Lubath. Bath oils used in the tub leave it oily and can cause falls. Better to apply directly to the skin.
- Hypoallergenic skin emollients and moisturizers recommended by Dr. Tripp are Aveeno Lotion, Complex 15, Moisturel, and Pen Kera. Pen Kera is very hypoallergenic; it has no dyes, lanolin, or fragrance. Moisturel is also very pure.
- Nonhypoallergenic skin emollients and moisturizers include: Aquaphor, Curel Lotion, Eucerin, Keri Lotion, Lubriderm, Neutragena Norwegian Formula, and Nutraderm (lanolin-free).
- For very itchy, dry skin or rashes, try Prax Lotion (contains an anti-itch chemical) or Sarna Lotion; medicated; no prescription required.
- For dry skin with thick scaling, use emollients containing urea, lactate, or salicylic acid, which cause a peeling of the skin by breaking up the dead skin and causing it to come off. They also smooth and soften thick, rough, or scaly skin. Try Aquacare HP, Eucerin, and Nutraplus, all available in both cream and lotion form; Epilyt Lotion, a new product; and Lacticare.

- Avoid use of fabric softener sheets, which can cause contact dermatitis; try a liquid softener or none at all.
- Before swimming, use a moistener on your skin. For ocean swimming, use a moisturizer containing a sunscreen with a #15 Sun Protection Factor (SPF), such as Nivea lotion.

TIPS FOR TAKING MEDICATIONS

- Swallow some water to lubricate your mouth and throat before putting a pill or capsule in the mouth.
- Put the pill or capsule as far back on your tongue as possible.
- Drink water from an empty soda bottle or similar bottle, keeping the lips on the bottle as you drink. This sets up a sucking action that makes the pill go down more easily.
- Stand up or sit as upright as possible to swallow medicine; this allows gravity to help get the medicine down.
- Wash medicine down with at least four ounces of water. If possible, drink another half glass of water, five minutes later.
- Stay in upright position for at least two or three minutes.
- If you are taking a pill at bedtime, do it before getting ready for bed, not before getting into bed.
- If the pill is stuck, eat several bites of a soft food, such as bread or bananas, then drink some water. The bulk will help push the pill downward. Try to avoid breaking tablets in half, since the ragged edges increase the likelihood of sticking.
- Immediately after taking a liquid medication, rinse your mouth with water to reduce the acidity from the medication, thus preventing possible mouth ulcers from forming.
- Metamucil should not be taken within two hours of any other medication. It may interfere with drug absorption.

PRESURGERY CAVEATS

This material is not part of anything previously published in *The Moisture Seekers Newsletter*. The information was prepared by Alan Rachleff, M.D., whose specialty is anesthesiology.

- Make sure that, *prior to your surgery,* each of the doctors involved in your care is aware that you have Sjögren's syndrome. Bring literature on Sjögren's syndrome with you when you go to the doctor and also to the hospital.
- Take a copy of the following information regarding anesthesia with you, and make sure you discuss each of these points preoperatively with all of the doctors and nurses involved in your care.

(1) Normally, patients undergoing general anesthesia require drugs preoperatively to reduce salivation, for example, atropine or scopolamine. These should be omitted in patients with Sjögren's syndrome. Antihistamines have a nonspecific sedative effect and are used for this purpose; they also tend to dry oral and nasal secretions. Other drugs, such as Valium or Compazine and their related compounds, should be used instead for their sedative properties.

(2) Probably the area of greatest concern is diminished tear production. Anesthesiologists often lubricate patients' eyes with petrolatum-based compounds and then tape them closed to prevent inadvertent abrasion. This would seem to be critical in those with Sjögren's syndrome.

(3) The anesthesiologist should be made aware of any joint pains or limited movement, particularly of the neck or jaw. If these pose severe problems, he may suggest greater safety in the choice of a block anesthetic, such as spinal or epidural, or a local anesthetic in the operative area, as opposed to general anesthesia.

(4) People nervous about being "wide awake" while being operated on are usually given sedative medication to doze lightly through the procedure. If this is applicable, suggest to the anesthesiologist that you bring your own artificial tears, if they are the most comfortable for you, and instruct him or her how frequently to instill them.

TRAVEL TIPS

Plane:

The relative humidity in an airplane is very low; therefore, it is important to fortify yourself with liquids and moisturizers.

Nose:
- Apply Borofax or Vaseline to the edges of nostrils. If you have a stuffed nose, use your medication before the plane takes off.
- Spray saline solution, such as Ayr, Nasal, Ocean, or Salinex, into your nose frequently during the trip.

Eyes:
- If you have moisture chamber glasses, make sure to wear them during the entire plane trip. If you don't, you might want to take either a sleep mask or swim or ski goggles to preserve the moisture in your eyes, at least while dozing.
- Use your artificial tears more frequently than you usually do.
- You might want to use a preservative-free emollient, such as many people use at night, for example, Akwa Tears, Duolube, Refresh P.M., or a more viscous eye drop for a plane trip.
- If your eyes hurt, ask the flight attendant for a hot washcloth to put over your eyes. This is particularly important for people with blepharitis. It's a good idea to keep a clean washcloth with you. Ask the flight attendant for a plastic cup, place your washcloth in it, have the attendant put a little hot water in it, and cover the container with another glass, so that the water and heat can permeate the cloth. SS patients who do not have blepharitis may find a washcloth that has been dipped in ice water soothing.

Mouth:
- Take a supply of sugarless gum or candy to suck and keep your mouth moist.
- Ask the flight attendant for a cup with a few ice cubes, and suck these to stimulate salivary secretions and provide moisture from the melting ice.

Skin:
- Carry a small tube of moisturizing cream, such as Aquacare HP, Carmol, or Nutraplus, to apply to your hands.

Car, train, or bus:
For prolonged travel, most of the information for plane travel can be adapted to travel on the road, particularly if you are a passenger.

- If you are driving, make sure you have a squirt bottle of water with a flip top cap, so that you can take frequent sips of water. Keep a can or squirt bottle of artificial saliva available.
- Pull over to the side of the road and use your eye drops *before* your eyes start to hurt.
- If you are driving, don't use eye ointment, because it causes blurring.
- Use one of the special containers mentioned above to keep your preservative-free eye drops cold enough to prevent bacterial growth.

Walking, hiking:
- Protect your eyes from dust, dirt, and wind with moisture chamber glasses.
- Wear tinted glasses and broad-brimmed hat to protect eyes from the sun.
- Use a sun screen with an SPF of at least 15 to protect your skin.

Smokefree Travel Guide:
This includes state-by-state listings, ranging from major hotel and restaurant chains with space reserved for nonsmokers, to bed and breakfast inns and cafes that maintain a totally smokefree environment. Copies can be ordered by sending a check for $12.95 to:

Nonsmokers' Rights
P. O. Box 668
Berkeley, CA 94701

Appendices

Appendix A

Glossary

achlorhydria: Gastric acid deficiency.

acne rosacea: Skin condition characterized by red nose and redness in other parts of the body.

adenopathy: A swelling of the lymph nodes. In Sjögren's syndrome, this usually occurs in the neck and jaw region.

alopecia: Hair loss.

alveoli: Air sacs of the lungs.

amylase: An enzyme present in saliva; another form of amylase is produced by the pancreas.

angular cheilitis: Sores at the corners of the mouth (angles of the lips).

antibody: Substance in the blood that is normally made in response to infection.

antifungal: Antagonistic (resisting) to fungi.

antigen(s): A chemical substance that provokes the production of antibody. In tetanus vaccination, for example, tetanus is the antigen injected to produce antibodies and hence protective immunity to tetanus.

antimalarial drugs: Quinine derivative drugs, which were first developed to treat malaria.

antispasmodic drugs: Medications that quiet spasms. Usually used in reference to the gastrointestinal tract.

arteriole: A very small artery.

ascites: An abnormal fluid that collects in the abdomen due to certain liver and other disorders.

atrophy: A thinning of the surface; a form of wasting.

autoantibody: Antibody that attacks the body's own tissues and organs as if they were foreign.

autoimmunity: Autoimmune disease is a state in which the body inappropriately produces antibody against its own tissues. In autoimmunity, the antigens are components of one's own body.

basal (resting) rate: Unstimulated (used in reference to both tears and salivary flow).

bolus: A morsel of food, already chewed, ready to be swallowed.

bronchi: Branches of the trachea.

buffer: A mixture of acid or base that, when added to a solution, enables the solution to resist changes in the pH that would otherwise occur when acid or alkali were added to it.

CAH: Chronic active hepatitis.

calcification: A process in which tissue or noncellular material in the body becomes hardened as the result of deposits of insoluble salts of calcium.

candidiasis: Moniliasis. A condition due to an overgrowth of the yeast (fungus) Candida.

cariostatic: Having the ability to help prevent dental caries.

celiac disease: Gluten intolerance.

CHB (congenital heart block): A dysfunction of the rate/rhythm conduction system in the fetal or infant heart.

CNS: The central nervous system (involving the brain and spinal cord).

connective tissue disease: A disorder marked by inflammation of the connective tissue (joints, skin, muscles) in multiple areas. In most instances, connective tissue diseases are associated with autoimmunity. Fifty percent of Sjögren's patients have connective tissue disorders.

cornea: The cornea is the clear "watch crystal" structure covering the pupil and iris (colored portion of the eye). It is composed of a number of vital layers, all of which are functionally important. The surface layer or epithelium is covered by the tears, which lubricate and protect the surface.

corticosteroid (steroid, cortisone): A hormone produced by the adrenal cortex gland. Natural adrenal gland hormones have powerful anti-inflammatory activity and are often used in the treatment of *severe* inflammation affecting vital organs. The multiple side effects of corticosteroids should markedly curtail their use in mild disorders.

cryoglobulins: Specific protein complexes circulating in the blood that are precipitated during cold.

cryptogenic cirrhosis (CC): Liver disease of unknown etiology (origin) with no history of alcoholism or previous acute hepatitis.

diuretics: Medications that increase the body's ability to rid itself of fluids.

double blind study: One in which neither the physician nor the patients being treated know whether patients are receiving the active ingredient being tested or a placebo (an inactive substance).

dysorexia: Impaired or deranged appetite.

dysphagia: Difficulty in swallowing. In Sjögren's syndrome, this may be attributable to several causes, among them decreased saliva, infiltration of the glands at the esophageal mucosa, or esophageal webbing.

dyspnea: Air hunger resulting in labored or difficult breathing, sometimes accompanied by pain.

ecchymosis: A purplish patch caused by oozing of blood into the skin; ecchymoses differ from petechia in size.

edema: Swelling caused by retention of fluid.

ELISA (enzyme-linked immunosorbent assay): A very sensitive blood test for detecting the presence of autoantibodies.

epistaxis: Nosebleed or hemorrhaging from the nose, which may be caused by dryness of the nasal mucous membrane in Sjögren's syndrome.

erythema: A medical term for a red color, usually associated with increased blood flow to an inflamed area, often the skin.

erythrocyte: Red blood cell.

esophagus: A canal (narrow tube) with muscular walls allowing passage of food from the pharynx or end of the mouth to the stomach.

ESR: Erythrocyte sedimentation rate. Measures the speed at which a column of bloods settles.

etiology: The cause(s) of a disease.

Eustachian tube: The tube running from the back of the nose to the middle ear.

exocrine glands: Glands that secrete mucus.

exocrinopathy: Disease related to the exocrine glands.

fibrosis: Abnormal formation of fibrous tissue.

fissure: A crack in the tissue surface (skin, tongue, etc.).

fluorescein stain: A dye that stains areas of the eye surface in which cells have been lost.

gastritis: Stomach inflammation.

genetic factors: Traits inherited from parents, grandparents, etc.

gingiva: The gums.

gingivitis: Inflammation of the gums.

granuloma: A nodular, inflammatory lesion.

HLA: Human lymphocyte antigens. A group of genes that govern the ability of lymphocytes, such as T-cells and B-cells, to respond to foreign and self substances.

idiopathic: Of unknown cause.

immunogenetics: The study of genetic factors that control the immune response.

immunoglobulins (gamma globulins): The protein fraction of serum responsible for antibody activity. Measurement of serum immunoglobulin levels can serve as a guide to disease activity in some patients with Sjögren's syndrome.

immunomodulators: Medications that affect the body's immune system.

immunosuppressive agents: A class of drugs that interferes with the function of cells that compose the immune system (see lymphocytes). Corticosteroids are immunosuppressive. Drugs used in the chemotherapy of malignant disease and in the prevention of transplant rejection are generally immunosuppressive and occasionally are used to treat severe autoimmune disease.

incisal: Cutting edge (of a tooth).

interstitial: Supporting structure in the substance of an organ or tissues.

interstitial nephritis: Inflammation of the connective tissue of the kidney, usually resulting in mild kidney disease characterized by frequent urination. Interstitial nephritis may be associated with Sjögren's syndrome.

intraoral: Inside the mouth.

KCS (keratoconjunctivitis sicca): This condition, also called dry eye, most frequently occurs in women in their forties and fifties. If associated with a dry mouth and/or rheumatoid arthritis, the condition is then referred to as Sjögren's syndrome.

lacrimal: Relating to the tears.

lacrimal glands: Two types of glands produce the essential fluid. Smaller accessory glands are found in the eyelid tissue and produce our "minute-to-minute" tear needs. The main lacrimal glands, located just inside the bony tissue surrounding the eye, can produce large amounts of tears.

Lacrisert: A small pellet, which is placed between the lower eyelid and eyeball once to twice daily. The pellet slowly disolves. Artificial tears are generally needed, also. Blurred vision is a commonly noted side effect.

larynx: Voice box.

latent: Not manifest, but potentially discernible.

lip biopsy: Incision of approximately two centimeters on inside surface of lower lip and excision of some of the minor salivary glands for microscopic examination and analysis.

lymph: A fluid collected from the tissues throughout the body, flowing through the lymph nodes, and eventually added to the circulating blood.

lymphocyte: A type of white blood cell concerned with antibody production and its regulation. Collections of lymphocytes are seen in the salivary glands of Sjögren's patients.

lymphoma: A severe proliferation (increase) of abnormal (malignant) lymphocytes, manifested as cancer of the lymph glands. Although exceedingly rare, lymphoma occurring as a complication of severe Sjögren's syndrome has been identified occasionally by immunologists.

matrix: The section of the tooth enamel that holds calcium and phosphate minerals.

MCTD: Mixed connective tissue disease.

Meibomian glands: Fat-producing glands found in the eyelids that produce an essential component of tears.

mucin: Thinnest layer of the tear film; layer closest to the cornea.

mucolytic agents: Medications that tend to dissolve mucus. Most dry eye patients complain of excess mucous discharge. Some patients may benefit from these medications, if other tear film-enhancing drops are less than adequately effective.

necrosis: Tissue death.

nephritis: An inflammation of the kidneys.

nonsteroidal anti-inflammatory drugs (NSAIDS): Chemical derivatives of acetylsalicylic acid (aspirin), which generally cause fewer side effects (e.g., heartburn), contain no cortisone, and are used to treat joint pains that occur in rheumatoid arthritis and other connective tissue disorders. Examples are: ibuprofen (Motrin), indomethacin (Indocin), sulindac (Clinoril), and piroxicam (Feldene).

nonspecific: Caused by other diseases or multiple factors.

olfactory: Relating to the sense of smell.

ophthalmologist: A physician who specializes in diseases and surgery of the eye.

oral mucosa: The lining (mucous membrane) of the mouth.

oral soft tissue: Tongue, mucous lining of the cheeks, and lips.

otitis: Inflammation of the ear, which may be marked by pain, fever, abnormalities of hearing, deafness, tinnitus, and vertigo. In

Sjögren's syndrome, blockage at Eustachian tubes due to infection can lead to conduction deafness and chronic otitis.

otolaryngologist: Physician specializing in ear, nose, and throat disorders.

palate biopsy: A punch biopsy near the junction of the hard and soft palates to sample the minor salivary glands in that region.

palpable: Perceptible to touch.

parasympathetic nervous system: The part of the autonomic nervous system whose functions include constriction of the pupils of the eyes, slowing of the heartbeat, and stimulation of certain digestive glands. These nerves originate in the midbrain, the hindbrain, and the sacral region of the spinal cord; impulses are mediated by acetylcholine.

parotid gland flow: An empirical, quantitative measure of the amount of saliva produced over a certain period of time. Normal parotid gland flow rate is 1.5 ml/min. In Sjögren's syndrome, flow rate is approximately .5 ml/min., with diminution of flow rate correlating inversely with severity of disease.

parotid glands: One of the three pairs of major salivary glands. They are located in front of the ear.

PBC: Primary biliary cirrhosis (an impairment of bile excretion secondary to liver inflammation and scarring).

perforation: A hole.

pericarditis: Inflammation of the lining of the heart.

periodontitis: Inflammation of the tissues surrounding and supporting the teeth.

peripheral nerves: Those outside the central nervous system.

petechia: A small, pinpoint, nonraised, perfectly round, purplish-red spot, caused by intradermal or submucosal hemorrhaging.

pharynx: Throat.

placebo: An inactive substance used as a "dummy" medication.

plaque: A thin, sticky film that builds up on the teeth, trapping harmful bacteria.

plasma: The fluid portion of the circulating blood.

pleurisy: Inflammation of the pleura (membrane surrounding the lungs and lining the walls of the rib cavity).

PM (polymyositis): A connective tissue disorder characterized by muscle pain and severe weakness secondary to inflammation in the major voluntary muscles.

psoralen: A drug administered topically or orally for the treatment of vitiligo (white skin patches caused by loss of pigment).

puncta: Small "holes" in the eyelids that normally drain tears. Patients with severe dry eye benefit from punctal closure, which allows maximal tear preservation.

purpura: A condition characterized by hemorrhage into the skin, appearing as crops of petechiae (very small red spots).

RA (rheumatoid arthritis): A form of arthritis characterized by inflammation of the joints, stiffness, swelling, cartilaginous hypertrophy, and pain.

radioactive isotope: Radioactive material used in diagnostic tests.

radionuclide studies: The technique in which radioactive isotopes, such as radiolabeled human serum albumin, are injected into an organ. A gamma scintillation camera, coupled with a digital computer system and cathode ray display, can read the radioactive emissions. Areas of perfusion will show marked radiographic emissions; areas of obstruction will show no activity.

Raynaud's phenomenon: Painful blanching of the fingertips on exposure to cold. This may be seen alone or in association with a connective tissue disease.

reflux: A regurgitation due to the return of gas, fluid, or small amount of food from the stomach.

renal: Relating to the kidneys.

RF: Rheumatoid factor. An autoantibody whose presence in the blood usually indicates autoimmune activity.

rheumatologist: A physician skilled in the diagnosis and treatment of rheumatic conditions.

rose bengal staining: A dye that stains abnormal or sick cells on the surface of the eye. This diagnostic dye allows the ophthalmologist to follow the treatment of dry eye.

salicylates: Aspirinlike drugs. (See nonsteroidal anti-inflammatory drugs).

salivary scintigraphy: Measurement of salivary gland function through injection of radioactive material.

sarcoidosis (Boeck's disease): A systemic disease with granulomatous (nodular, inflammatory) lesions involving the lungs and, on occasion, the salivary glands, with resulting fibrosis.

Schirmer test: The standard objective test to diagnose dry eye. Small pieces of filter paper are placed between the lower eyelid and eyeball and soak tears for five minutes. The value obtained is a rough estimation of tear production in relative terms. Lower values are consistent with dry eye. It is important to emphasize that no single test can be considered diagnostic unless the condition is severe.

scleroderma: A connective tissue disorder characterized by thickening and hardening of the skin. Sometimes internal organs (intestines, kidneys) are affected, causing bowel irregularity and high blood pressure.

serum: The fluid portion of the blood (obtained after removal of the fibrin clot and blood cells), distinguished from the plasma in the circulation blood.

sialochemistry: Measuring the constituents in saliva.

sialography: X-ray examination of the salivary duct system by use of liquid contrast medium. Radiologically sensitive dye is placed into the duct system, serving to outline the ductal system clearly.

signs: Changes that can be seen or measured.

Sjögren's antibodies: Abnormal antibodies found in the sera of Sjögren's syndrome patients. These antibodies react with the extracts of certain cells, and a test based on this principle can be helpful in the diagnosis of Sjögren's.

Sjögren's syndrome: A symptom complex of dry eyes, dry mouth, and other mucous membranes associated with inflammation in the lacrimal and/or salivary glands. It can occur alone (50%) or in association with a connective tissue disease.

SLE (systemic lupus erythematosus): An inflammatory connective tissue disease.

SS-A: Sjögren's syndrome-associated antigen A (anti-Ro).

SS-B: Sjögren's syndrome-associated antigen B (anti-La).

steatorrhea: Greasy stools (passage of large amounts of fat in the feces, as occurs in pancreatic disease and the malabsorption syndromes).

steroids: Cortisone-derivative medications.

sublingual glands: One of the three pairs of major salivary glands. They are located in the floor of the mouth, under the tongue.

submandibular glands: One of the three pairs of major salivary glands. They are located below the lower jaw.

symptoms: Changes patients feel.

systemic: Any process that involves multiple organ systems throughout the body.

thrush: A form of candidiasis. Infection of the oral tissues with *Candida albicans.*

thryoiditis: A disease in which autoantibodies cause immune system cells (lymphocytes) to destroy the thryoid gland.

titer: Test showing strength or concentration of a particular volume of a solution. Usually used to refer to amounts of antibody present.

TMJ (temporomandibular joint): The joint of the lower jaw where the "ball-and-socket" arrangement is formed by the condyle of the lower jaw (the ball) and the fossa of the temporal bone (the socket). The joint space is filled with synovial or lubricating fluid. This joint and surrounding synovial tissues may become inflamed, if rheumatoid arthritis accompanies Sjögren's syndrome and involves this joint.

trachea: Windpipe.

tracheobronchial tree: The windpipe and the two bronchi into which it subdivides.

urticaria: Hives.

vasculitis: Inflammation of a blood vessel.

venule: A very small vein.

viscera: The organs of the digestive, respiratory, urogenital, and endocrine systems, as well as the spleen, heart, and great vessels (blood and lymph ducts).

vitiligo: White patches on the skin due to loss of pigment.

xerostomia: Dryness of the mouth caused by the arresting of normal salivary secretions. It occurs in diabetes, drug therapy, radiation therapy, and Sjögren's syndrome.

xylitol: A sweetening agent with cariostatic properties.

Appendix B

Moisture Chamber Eyeglasses

Kenneth Berk, O.D.
Bonnie A. Gustafsson

Maintaining sufficient tears for adequate lubrication of the eye is very important for the person who has dry eyes. For many patients, artificial tear solutions are not enough. These patients may benefit from moisture chamber eyeglasses, in addition to tear substitutes.

By preventing evaporation of existing tears and of instilled solutions, moisture chambers enhance patient comfort and reduce irritation from air currents, fumes, and other elements.

The following instructions are a guide for the optician who wishes to make moisture chamber eyeglasses for his patients.

HOW MOISTURE CHAMBER EYEGLASSES ARE MADE

Moisture chambers must be custom-fitted accurately for each patient. Several adjustments may be necessary. If the patient already wears eyeglasses, moisture chambers are fitted over the frame of these glasses. (Some considerations regarding frame style are discussed below.) If the patient does not wear glasses to improve vision, moisture chamber glasses are made with frames containing nonpowered lenses.

After experiments with several designs and materials, the following method has proven the most manageable and effective (see corresponding figures):

(1) The frame should be of zyl material, with an eye size of between 50 and 58 mm. The frame shape should have gentle curves, without sharp angles. Position is not critical. The temple may be mounted high, low, or intermediate. All adjustments to the frame front and front of the temples must be made before the vinyl is secured to the frame. The vinyl cannot be heated, since it would buckle and become distorted.

(2) The rear shelf of the eyewire (the area behind the groove) should be a minimum width of 1 mm. Because this is the area to which the vinyl will be glued, it must be sufficient for firm bonding.

(3) The vinyl used in the moisture chambers should be approximately .4 to .5 mm. thick. It should be flexible, similar to the vinyl used in upholstery covering. Cut a rectangular piece, measuring about 6 cm. x 14 cm.

(4) Roll vinyl into an open cylinder.

(5) Insert the cylinder into the eyewire, so that the open position is adjacent to the nose pad area, with approximately 1 cm. or less protruding through the front of the frame. The cylinder may be held in this position by inserting spring-loaded clothespins from the front of the frame. Six to eight clothespins, closely spaced, usually are adequate for an average-size frame.

(6) Insert liquid Krazy-Glu (cyanoacetate) at point A. The cement should run around the full circumference of the rear of the eyewire, where it abuts the vinyl. After the cement has cured, remove the clothespins and check the strength of the cement joint by tugging on the vinyl. If necessary, any weak areas can now be glued from the back of the eyewire, without further clamping. When the bond is firm and continuous, the vinyl should be cut at point B (the rear of the groove) with either a sharp X-Acto knife, a Mototool, or an equivalent.

(7) After the vinyl to the front of the groove is peeled away, the groove should be cleaned of any excess glue that may have seeped to the front of the eyewire. The vinyl adjacent to the groove should be trimmed as close as possible to align it with the groove.

(8) Now there should be an open cylinder of vinyl attached

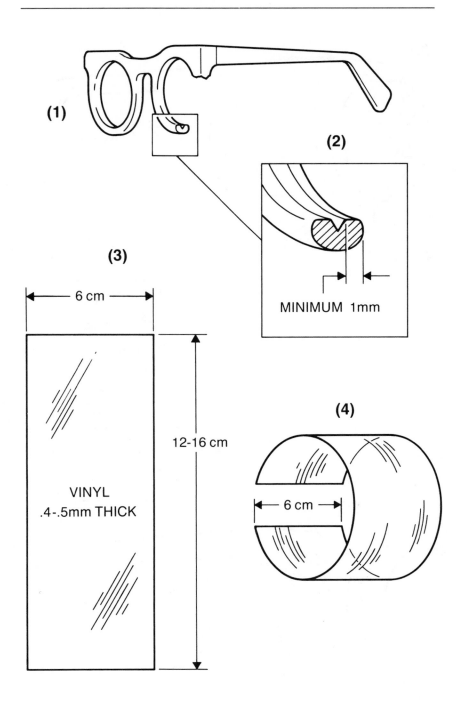

(1)

(2)

MINIMUM 1mm

(3)

← 6 cm →

12-16 cm

VINYL
.4-.5mm THICK

(4)

← 6 cm →

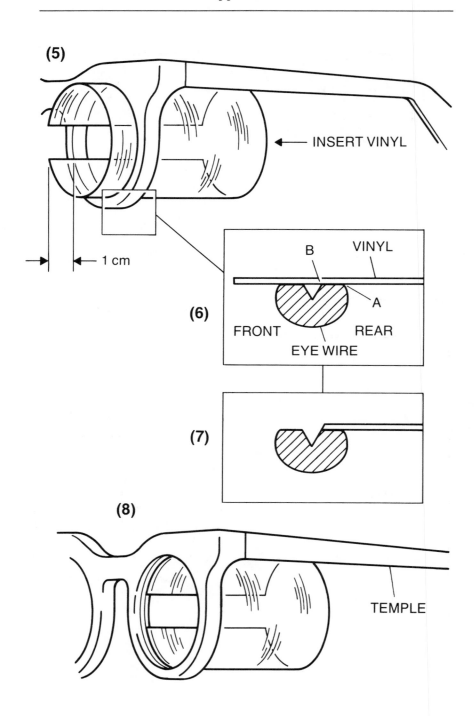

(5)

← INSERT VINYL

1 cm

(6)

B   VINYL

A

FRONT   REAR

EYE WIRE

(7)

(8)

TEMPLE

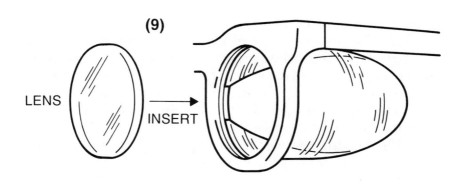

(9)

LENS → INSERT

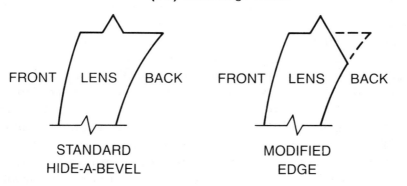

(10) Lens Edge Detail

FRONT | LENS | BACK

STANDARD
HIDE-A-BEVEL

FRONT | LENS | BACK

MODIFIED
EDGE

(11) Finished/Inserted Edge Detail

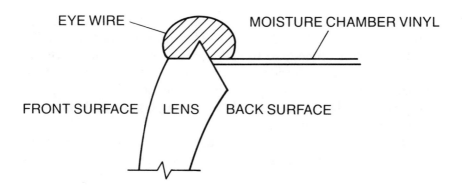

EYE WIRE — MOISTURE CHAMBER VINYL

FRONT SURFACE | LENS | BACK SURFACE

to the rear of the eyewire.

(9) The vinyl should be trimmed with sharp scissors or cuticle scissors, so that before fitting the patient, the final shape of the vinyl approximates the shape of the leather shields on Bausch & Lomb Glacier Glasses. However, do not cut away too much material. Ample vinyl is needed to allow the shield to be trimmed to fit the patient's facial contours.

(10) Plastic lenses must be used, preferably scratch-resistant plastic. Since the frame containing the vinyl cannot be heated for lens insertion or adjustment, the lens must be trimmed for a snap-in fit from the front of the frame. Ideally, the lens should be finished with a full V-bevel. However, a Hide-a-Bevel edge may be modified by grinding away the rear of the lens to approximate a V-bevel.

(11) If all goes well, the lens will snap into place without interfering with the vinyl chamber. The frame may even be re-glazed in the future by removing the original lens through the front of the frame. If the moisture chambers are damaged, they may be peeled away from the frame. The frame may be cleaned, sanded, filed, and polished, and a replacement vinyl chamber may be attached in the manner described above. In time, vinyl will age, discolor, and crack due to oxidation, ultraviolet rays, perspiration, and makeup. How long the chambers will last varies from patient to patient, but they can usually be replaced.

FINAL FITTING

In the first step of the final fitting, the patient attempts to place the glasses gently on the face. The fitter observes where the vinyl must be trimmed, so that the glasses will rest in a normal position. To avoid accidental loss of too much vinyl, small amounts are cut away during trimming. Ideally, when trimming is complete, the glasses should sit in a normal, comfortable position on the face, nose, and ears.

The edge of the moisture chamber should come within 1 mm. to 2 mm. of the skin surface, not pressing into the skin. This not only prevents the vinyl from leaving marks on the skin, but also helps keep the vinyl clean. The object is not to create a hermetic seal, which would cause the lenses to fog. Although some fogging is unavoidable, the purpose of the moisture chamber is to prevent excessive air currents from evaporating available tears. If excessive fogging occurs, the vinyl may be trimmed slightly to allow adequate ventilation.

After the chambers are trimmed to the optimum fit, a moderately coarse carborundum paper or its equivalent is used to smooth the edge of the vinyl.

ADDITIONAL INFORMATION AND SUGGESTIONS

Although the weight added to the frame by the amount of vinyl is extremely small, some patients are sensitive enough to notice it.

The moisture chambers and glasses are cleaned with any standard spray cleaner and a fresh facial tissue.

Before cementing to the frame, the vinyl for moisture chamber sunglasses may be dyed in standard dye tanks to approximate the color of the frame or the lenses. Because the vinyl may wrinkle, it should be immersed in the dye for only seconds at at time and immediately cooled with rinse water. For darker colors, immerse the vinyl repeatedly.

The temples should not be closed over the moisture chambers; otherwise, permanent distortion of the chambers may result. Because the temples should never be folded, a small cigar box, which may be lined, upholstered, or decorated in other ways, makes the best carrying case.

Because moisture chambers provide benefits only while being worn, they should be worn continually or as needed. This also avoids wear and tear on the glasses caused by constantly taking them on and off.

Moisture chamber glasses are *not* substitutes for artificial tear solutions. They prolong the effect of tear solutions by preventing evaporation.

Appendix C

The Sjögren's Syndrome Foundation Inc.

The letters SSF, well known today to Sjögren's syndrome patients and the doctors who treat them, stand for the Sjögren's Syndrome Foundation Inc. The Foundation, which had its birth in December, 1983, at the Long Island Jewish Medical Center (LIJMC), New Hyde Park, NY, came into this world as "The Moisture Seekers." In 1985, when the Foundation was formally incorporated, the Board of Directors voted to use the name of the disease as the official name of the organization, so that both the public and medical professionals would be able to identify us immediately (if they knew what Sjögren's syndrome was).

Dolores Sciubba, wife of Dr. James J. Sciubba, the first chairman of our Medical Advisory Board, appreciated my reluctance to give up the name "Moisture Seekers," which I felt so aptly described our purpose. Thanks to her suggestion, that name was retained for our monthly newsletter.

Despite the fact that public awareness of Sjögren's syndrome is on the increase, "Sjögren's" is still a very difficult name to pronounce, and we receive many calls from people who say, "Is this the S-j-(spelling out each letter)?" The pronunciation of Dr. Sjögren's name is "SHOW-gren."

DOING SOMETHING POSITIVE

Like most SS sufferers, I, too, was a lonely, desperate patient, both before my diagnosis and immediately thereafter. When I was diagnosed in 1982, there was no self-help group for SS patients, and I didn't know any other patients. During my frequent visits to LIJMC, I became friendly with Flo Goldberg, a doctor's secretary, who seemed to have problems similar to mine. Before the doctors had figured out what she had, I told her, "I think you have what I have." And she did.

At this time (summer of 1983), I was feeling particularly desperate. Dr. Steven Carsons, my immunologist, told me, "Elaine, you either have to go for help or do something positive." Flo and I decided to do something positive. Flo, who also had rheumatoid arthritis, contacted the Arthritis Foundation in New York City about starting a self-help group at LIJMC. She was turned down, because her primary concern was rheumatoid arthritis, and LIJMC was too close to other arthritis self-help groups in the vicinity.

I refused to give up. I informed the Arthritis Foundation that what I really wanted was a Sjögren's syndrome group. Okay, they said, but a leader must be trained, and their training course had just ended; I would have to wait until spring. But I was persistent. I impressed upon them all the community work I had done, courses I had taken in group dynamics, etc., and was sent on to Carol Eisman, then associated with the New York City Self-Help Clearinghouse, for final approval and a private training session. (Carol is now in Los Angeles.)

I was excited. Despite feeling like something "the cat wouldn't even want to drag out of the garbage can," I had important work to do and could not allow myself to give in to all the pain and fatigue. I had to pace myself. And I did.

My visits to the three doctors at LIJMC responsible for my SS care must have thrown their schedules completely off, because, as I discussed my ideas with them, they too became excited, very supportive, and involved in starting a Sjögren's syndrome mutual-aid group. These three doctors, Dr. Steven Carsons, Dr. James J. Sciubba, and Dr. Ira Udell (a cornea specialist) did more than just talk to me about the group. They enlisted the interest and support of colleagues and urged them to help by serving on our Medical Advisory Board. We were on our way.

The members of our Medical Advisory Board, at the time that the Moisture Seekers was formed, were: Chairman, James J. Sciubba, D.M.D., Ph.D., Steven Carsons, M.D., Herbert S. Diamond, M.D., Robert A. Greenwald, M.D., Howard Kerpen, M.D., Ira J. Udell, M.D., and Howard Weiss, M.D. We are most grateful to each of them for their counsel and guidance. The members of the Medical Advisory Board for 1989, together with their academic affiliations, are listed at the end of this appendix.

Dr. Sciubba, Chairman of the Department of Dentistry at LIJMC, arranged for a meeting room and informed his other SS patients about our group. The New York Chapter of the Arthritis Foundation (AF) gave us seed money for our first two mailings. They also put me in touch with the Long Island Chapter of the AF. Chickie Goldstein, Medical Director, and Frances Mason, Self-Help Coordinator of the New York Chapter, and Pat McAsey, Executive Director of the Long Island Chapter, have been wonderful consellors and supporters. Both groups, as well as the Patient Services Department at Arthritis Foundation headquarters in Atlanta, continue to help by referring their SS patient inquiries to us and by publicizing our symposium and local meetings.

At our first meeting in December, 1983, the small conference room (so that the room wouldn't look too empty, if only a few people showed up) that had been reserved was filled to overflowing. Fourteen frustrated patients and 11 family members attended. We decided to meet the following month—in a larger room. It was exciting. We were learning and sharing.

The following September, *The New York Times* printed my reply to a Jane Brody column about dry mouth. Thanks to the national and international circulation of *The Times,* inquiries started coming in from all over the country. The fall of 1984 also marked our first symposium, with Dr. Norman Talal as our guest speaker.

In April, 1984, the Long Island Weekly section of *The New York Times* carried an article about our self-help group. There is nothing that can equal a good story in print, regardless of how much more glamorous a TV or radio interview may seem. People can cut it out, photocopy it, and sent it to friends and relatives. And that is exactly what occurred as a result of that article. A woman in New York sent it to her friend in Los Angeles, because she remembered that her friend's daughter, who happened to be living in Seattle, had SS—and that was the start of our Seattle Chapter. And a doctor at the National Institutes of Health (NIH) told one of his "go-getter" patients about us—the start of our Washington, DC, Chapter.

In January, 1984, at our second meeting, it was decided to "pass the cup" to offset future mailing costs. And by our third meeting, attendees were so enthusiastic that they suggested we have membership dues. Our problem became an administrative one, since we were not yet incorporated and therefore could not get an organization bank account in New York State. Dr. Sciubba came to the rescue by helping obtain a special hospital account for our group until our incorporation in the summer of 1985.

THE MOISTURE SEEKERS NEWSLETTER

Our next big step forward came as a result of a meeting that had been arranged with some officers of the Lupus Foundation of America (LFA), when they were on Long Island. Although we had arranged the meeting to learn more about bylaws, chapters, etc., the most productive part of the meeting was that Fran Heims and I were very excited about the newsletter the LFA put out. We thought putting out a simple newsletter could serve a dual purpose—a report on the past meeting, as well as a notice for the coming meeting.

Fran, who is not an SS patient, offered to help edit the sheet.

She designed our first logo. I took the finished copy over to LIJMC, where Dr. Sciubba's secretary gave me permission to photocopy the 30 copies we needed for our first issue in May, 1984. Although Fran could not continue to help due to back surgery, our newsletter owes its birth to her help.

By October, 1984, we had expanded to a four-page, professionally printed newsletter. Once again, LIJMC came to our rescue and helped with the actual mailing. Bob Adams, a commercial artist and husband of one of our members, Laura Adams, offered to design a logo for us. This is now the familiar logo appearing on every issue of *The Moisture Seekers Newsletter.*

The next most wonderful thing that happened was that Bonnie Gustafsson joined the organization and offered her writing talent to do the monthly report on the speaker presentations at the LIJMC meetings. Bonnie currently works and lives in New Jersey. She manages to get to Long Island for the annual symposium, and we are all very grateful for her excellent reports on the symposium speakers.

The sorting and mailing of our newsletter was directed for two years by Marcella and Harry Dobrow. The current task of mailing 6,000 copies of *The Moisture Seekers Newsletter* to patients and doctors throughout the world has become too large to be handled without special equipment to take the computer-addressed mailing labels from strips and apply them to the newsletter. This must be done from a well equipped mail room.

PRO BONO SERVICES

Organizations such as ours are very dependent on personal friends and contacts for pro bono services. To Sherman Lawrence, Esq., we will be forever indebted for filing the papers necessary for our incorporation as a nonprofit organization in the State of New York.

We will never forget my dear friend Sylvan Gefen, recently departed, for his devoted and excellent service as the Foundation's accountant from its creation until he became critically ill late in 1988.

If you think filing a personal income tax is a bother, you should see the records and work necessary for nonprofit organizations such as ours.

Louise Gibson, our treasurer, not only efficiently records receipts and pays our bills, but she is very actively involved in all phases of the Foundation's daily activities, planning and development, membership services, and chapter relations.

Herb Harris, my dear husband, currently devotes the majority of his time to developing computer programs for the SSF, so that labels for newsletters can come out in zip code order, records of new members for each chapter can be sent to the proper leaders, renewal notices can go out, special letters can be sent to a targeted section of our mailing list, etc.

SJOGREN'S SYNDROME SYMPOSIUM

"Living with Sjögren's, Day-to-Day With a Chronic Disease" is the subtitle of our annual symposium. It aptly describes the focus of the program, which is to bring to patients and interested health professionals the latest news concerning treatment and practical ways of dealing with the various aspects of the disease.

The program usually consists of a guest speaker noted for his work related to the diagnosis or treatment of a particular aspect of Sjögren's syndrome. The distinguished guest speakers have been: 1984, Dr. Norman Talal; 1985, Dr. Harry Spiera; 1986, Dr. Philip Fox; 1987, Dr. Jan U. Prause; and 1988, Dr. Haralampos Moutsopoulos. In addition to guest speakers, the program has also had a Resource Panel of specialists, usually in rheumatology or immunology, ophthalmology, and dentistry.

The 1988 symposium had for the first time a separate morning session, "Living with Sjögren's in the Family," a discussion of the psychological implications of living with a chronic illness. The discussion was led by Dr. Robert Phillips, a clinical psychologist who, as Director of the Center for Coping with Chronic Conditions, is well known for his work with patients who have illnesses for which there is at present no cure.

Although the symposium presentations are reported in *The Moisture Seekers Newsletter,* and tapes of the program are also available, the requests from our members in various parts of the country for similar programs closer to their home base has prompted the Board of Directors to consider holding the symposium in a different city each year.

CHAPTER DEVELOPMENT

Growing is not all glorious, even if it is glamorous. The many chapters and contact leaders listed in each newsletter require much servicing—from the initial request to serve as an "arm" of the Foundation and, to some degree, forever after.

To Anita Shehi, who helped develop some excellent step-by-step procedures to be followed, and to Harriett Miller, who has succeeded Anita as Vice President for Chapter Development, we are particularly grateful for enabling the Foundation to reach out to more and more people. Harriett Miller has just arranged for some of our materials to be translated into Spanish for the benefit of our Latin American members. Vice President Laura Adams is handling the development of overseas affiliates.

A tremendous amount of work is necessary to service our chapters and to make certain that all activities conform with the Foundation's standards and bylaws and with the IRS regulations for nonprofit organizations. Our high standards have resulted in recognition by many "networking" organizations. The National Institute of Dental Research (NIDR), the Arthritis Foundation, health columnists, the American Academy of Ophthalmology (AAO), and the NIH Office of Public Health Information Clearinghouse (OPHIC) all refer SS patients to our Foundation for information and help on SS.

Increasing medical interest and awareness of Sjögren's syndrome is a most important function of the Foundation. The 1989 NIH Conference on "The Many Faces of Sjögren's Syndrome" was a direct result of testimony that Betsy Latiff, member of the

SSF Board of Directors, and I gave in 1987 before the National Commission on Orphan Diseases. Betsy is our liaison with the pharmaceutical industry, trying to encourage them to develop medications that will help our multitudinous problems. Joan Manny serves as our Washington and NIH liaison, representing us at conferences and meetings.

INTERNATIONAL AFFILIATES

In 1985, I received a call from Lyn Linse, a resident of Great Britain, who was in the United States visiting her family. She had heard of our existence from Biosonics, Inc. We corresponded regularly and, on her next visit to the United States, we met at JFK Airport in New York and discussed how Lyn could start a British affiliate of the SSF.

The British Sjögren's Syndrome Association (BSSA), which meets regularly, is the result of her efforts. Lyn and her husband are now living in Scotland, and Lyn, as soon as she is properly settled, plans to start a group there. Lyn still edits the excellent *BSSA Newsletter,* and we have reprinted some of its articles in *The Moisture Seekers Newsletter.*

As a result of my attending the First International Conference on Sjögren's Syndrome, which took place in May, 1986, in Copenhagen, overseas awareness and interest in the Sjogren's Syndrome Foundation was greatly increased. I personally was able to explain our needs as patients, including the inadequacies of many of the palliatives prescribed for SS, as well as our need for more information about our disease. Many of the doctors attending that conference not only have become members of the Foundation, but are actively helping us. Jan Prause (Denmark) and Harry Moutsopoulos (Greece) have been guest speakers at our annual symposia. Dr. Susumu Sugai of Japan heads his country's affiliate of the SSF, and he is planning to translate this handbook into Japanese.

Several of our overseas medical friends are working with their local patients to start SSF affiliates. Dr. Daniele Goldberg, who became our "French Connection" as a result of her work with Dr. Talal, took care of several of our members who wanted medical advice while visiting Paris, last winter, in addition to taking care of her own Parisian patients.

At the Second International Conference on Sjögren's Syndrome, held in Austin, TX, in October, 1988, under the chairmanship of Dr. Norman Talal, our national and international connections were strengthened and increased. Several of the doctors have promised to write articles for *The Moisture Seekers Newsletter* about the research they are doing. Doctors Jehudith and Yehuda Scharf have just completed their sabbatical and, now that they are back in Israel, are hoping to start an Israeli SSF connection.

Our Dutch affiliate, the Nationale Vereniging Sjögrenpatienten, was already in existence when Mr. H. Lissenberg, their president, contacted us about joining our international network, which they did in 1987. Ruth Borah, one of their members, attended our 1987 symposium. Ruth has kindly translated the minutes of their meetings into English.

NETWORKING WITH OTHER ORGANIZATIONS

In September, 1987, as President of the SSF, I was one of 160 self-help leaders chosen to attend Surgeon General Dr. Edward Koop's Conference on Self-Help. Several times, discussion centered on improving the credibility of a group and its recognition by medical professionals. I felt proud that our Foundation has encountered no such difficulties and that we have been recommended by medical professionals for the help we render our members.

This handbook is a perfect example of the cooperation that exists between doctors and our Foundation. Furthermore, the recently published medical textbook, *Sjögren's Syndrome: Clinical and Immunological Aspects,* edited by Dr. N. Talal, Dr. H. M. Moutsopoulos, and Dr. S. S. Kassan, contains a chapter, "The Patient's Perspective," written by SSF President and Founder

Elaine Harris. According to Dr. Talal, this contribution by a patient to a medical textbook is unique. It once again demonstrates
the high esteem that the medical experts on Sjögren's syndrome
have for the Foundation.

For a year now, we have been exhibiting our literature and
services at professional conferences, such as the American Rheu-
matism Association, now the Americal College of Rheumatology;
the American Academy of Ophthalmology; and the American
Dental Association (ADA) annual conferences. The excellence of
our exhibits (Barbara Henry and Anita Shehi received a first prize
for their exhibit at the 1987 ADA meeting in Las Vegas) and the
materials we distribute to patients are increasing medical awareness about SS and helping to keep the medical professsionals alert
to our needs.

The history of our Foundation would be incomplete without
mention of the National Organization for Rare Disorders
(NORD) and Abbey Meyers, their Executive Director. Abbey's
counsel in directing Betsy's and my efforts to persuade Boehringer-
Ingelheim to institute trials relating to bromhexine as a safe and
effective medication for SS has been invaluable. Her help in intro-
ducing us to the proper people in the Federal Drug Administration
(FDA) and Office for the Development of Orphan Drugs will never
be forgotten. NORD's annual meeting is a learning experience,
which I wish each of our chapter and contact leaders could attend.
It is an opportunity for sharing knowledge, learning new techniques, getting the latest information on how government actions
will affect our organization, and appreciating the problems of
other groups.

Connective tissue diseases, such as scleroderma, lupus, and
Raynaud's syndrome, not only affect SS patients, but have several
common manifestations. Networking among the organizations
representing these diseases is important. We share patients, information, and skills. Nancy and Harlan Hersey of the Scleroderma
Information Exchange not only put us in touch with other scleroderma groups, but have twice travelled from Rhode Island to Long
Island to videotape our symposium.

OFFICERS OF THE SJOGREN'S SYNDROME FOUNDATION

A history of the Foundation would not be complete without a list of our officers and Board of Directors at the time of incorporation in 1985. They were: President, Elaine K. Harris; Vice Presidents, Laura Adams and Stella Nadel; Secretary, Marveen Christie; Treasurer, Louise Gibson. Board of Directors: the preceding officers and Ethel Brown, Marcella Dobrow, Mary Dunphy, Bonnie Gustafsson, Helen Kay, and Fritzie Marsa. Each of them has played a role in our successful development.

For 1989, the Foundation officers will be: President, Elaine K. Harris; Vice Presidents, Laura Adams and Harriett Miller; Secretary, Gilda Kaback; Treasurer, Louise Gibson. Board of Directors: the preceding officers and Pidge Boyles, Mark Flapan, Ph.D., Bonnie Gustafsson, Barbara Henry, Betsy Latiff, Morton J. Levy, Joan Manny, and Sheldon Newman.

1989 MEDICAL ADVISORY BOARD

CHAIRMAN
Norman Talal, M.D.
Professor of Medicine and Microbiology
Head, Division of Clinical Immunology and Rheumatology
University of Texas Health Science Center at San Antonio and
Audie Murphy Memorial Veterans Administration Hospital
7703 Floyd Curl Drive
San Antonio, TX 78284

MEDICAL LIAISON TO BOARD OF DIRECTORS
Steven Carsons, M.D.
Assistant Professor of Medicine
Health Sciences Center
State University of New York at Stony Brook
Chief of Rheumatology, Clinical Immunology, and Allergy
Winthrop University Hospital
Mineola, NY 11501

MEDICAL ADVISORY BOARD MEMBERS

Troy E. Daniels, D.D.S., M.S.
Professor of Oral Medicine and Oral Pathology
Chairman of Oral Pathology
Director, Sjögren's Syndrome Clinic
School of Dentistry
University of California, San Francisco
San Francisco, CA 94143

Vincent P. deLuise, M.D.
Assistant Clinical Professor of Ophthalmology
University of Connecticut in Farmington
Adjunct Assistant Professor of Ophthalmology
Cornell University Medical College
Opticare Eye Health Center
87 Grandview Avenue
Waterbury, CT 06708

R. Linsy Farris, M.D.
Professor of Clinical Ophthalmology
College of Physicians and Surgeons
Columbia University
Attending Physician, Cornea and External Eye Disease
Edward S. Harkness Eye Institute
Columbia-Presbyterian Medical Center
Director of Opthalmology
Harlem Hospital Medical Center
635 West 165 Street
New York, NY 10032

Philip Fox, D.D.S.
Head, Clinical Studies Unit
National Institute of Dental Research
NIH, Building 10, Room 1B-21
Bethesda, MD 20892

Robert I. Fox, M.D., Ph.D.
Adjunct Assistant Member
Department of Basic and Clinical Research
Scripps Clinic and Research Foundation
10666 North Torrey Pines Road
La Jolla, CA 92037

Richard Furie, M.D.
Assistant Attending Physician, Hospital for Special Surgery
Assistant Professor of Medicine
Cornell University Medical College
Assistant Attending Physician
Division of Rheumatology and Clinical Immunology
North Shore University Hospital
300 Community Drive
Manhasset, NY 11030

Jeffrey Gilbard, M.D.
Associate Clinical Scientist, Eye Research Institute
Assistant Clinical Professor, Harvard Medical School
ERI, 20 Staniford Street
Boston, MA 02114

John S. Greenspan, B.D.S., Ph.D.
Professor and Acting Chairman, Department of Stomatology
School of Dentistry
University of California, San Francisco
San Francisco, CA 94143

Robert A. Greenwald, M.D.
Assistant Professor of Rheumatology,
Health Sciences Center
State University of New York at Stony Brook
Chief, Division of Rheumatology
Long Island Jewish Medical Center
New Hyde Park, NY 11042

Stuart S. Kassan, M.D.
Associate Clinical Professor of Medicine
University of Colorado
Medical Director, Rehabilitation Center
Lutheran Medical Center
4200 West Conejos Place
Denver, CO 80204

Irwin D. Mandel, D.D.S.
Professor of Dentistry
Director, Center for Clinical Research in Dentistry
School of Dental and Oral Surgery
Columbia University
630 West 168 Street
New York, NY 10032

Haralampos M. Moutsopoulos, M.D.
Professor and Chairman, Department of Internal Medicine
Medical School, University of Ioannina
45 332 Ioannina, GREECE

Roger Miles Rose, M.D.
Associate Professor of Otolaryngology-Head and Neck Surgery
New York University College of Medicine
Attending Physician, New York University Medical Center and
Lenox Hill Hospital
127 East 61 Street
New York, NY 10021

James J. Sciubba, D.M.D., Ph.D.
Professor of Oral Biology and Pathology
School of Dental Medicine
State University of New York
Chairman, Department of Dentistry
Long Island Jewish Medical Center
New Hyde Park, NY 11042

Harry Spiera. M.D.
Clinical Professor of Medicine
Chief, Division of Rheumatology
Mount Sinai Medical Center
1 Gustave Levy Place
New York, NY 10029

Ira J. Udell, M.D.
Assistant Professor of Ophthalmology
Health Sciences Center
State University of New York at Stony Brook
Physician-in-Charge, Cornea and External Eye Disease
Long Island Jewish Medical Center
New Hyde Park, NY 11042

John J. Willems, M.D.
Associate Clinical Professor
University of California, San Diego
Director, Vulvar Disease Clinic
Scripps Clinic and Research Foundation
10666 North Torrey Pines Road
La Jolla, CA 92037

The Sjogren's Syndrome Foundation has turned Sjögren's syndrome from a disease that hardly anyone had even heard about into one that is receiving increasing attention and help from medical professionals. To all the people who have helped us reach this stage, only some of whom have been specifically mentioned, my personal thanks and those of every Sjögren's syndrome patient. And to the patients, the public, the medical professionals, and the business organizations who would like to help us in our efforts, I invite your participation and financial support.

Elaine K. Harris

Index